Fiona Marshall is a freelance journalist and author. She writes regularly for the UK health and medical press.

By the same author

The Natural Way: Epilepsy

Your Child: Epilepsy

Coping Successfully with your Second Child

Coping with Postnatal Depression

Losing a Parent

NATURAL APHRODISIACS

Fiona Marshall

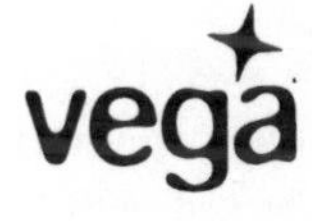

ISBN 1-84333-330-9

A catalogue record for this book is available from the British Library

Published in 2002 by
Vega
64 Brewery Road
London, N7 9NT

A member of **Chrysalis** Books plc

Visit our website at www.chrysalisbooks.co.uk

Cover design: Grade Design Consultants, London
Printed in Great Britain by Creative Print & Design Wales

A note from the publisher
Any information given in this book is not intended to be taken as a replacement for medical advice. Any person with a condition requiring medical attention should consult a qualified medical practitioner or suitable therapist.

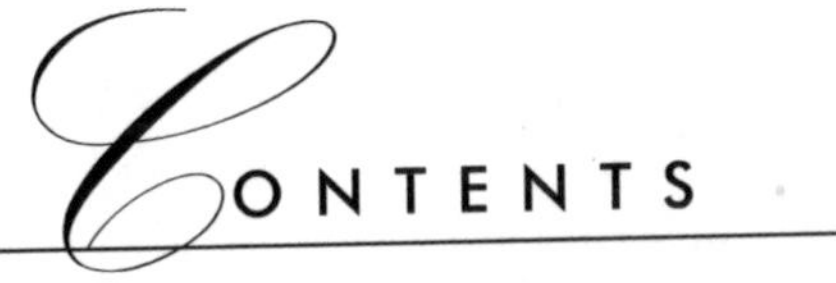

CONTENTS

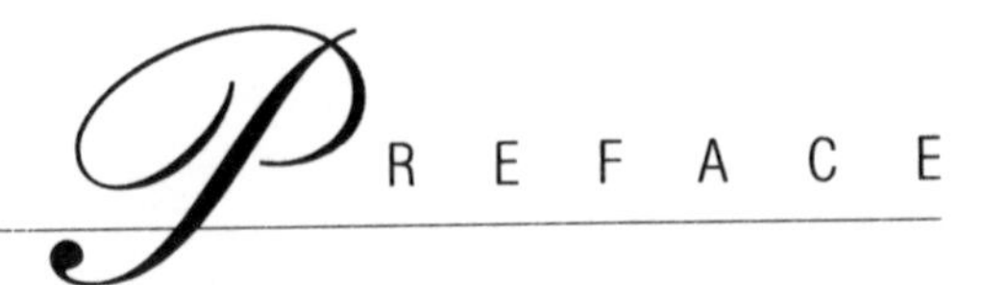

PREFACE

The drive to seek sexual satisfaction is as old as mankind. Rooted in compelling physical forces, and as vital as food for the survival of the species, sex is a creative way of expressing love, and may involve emotional and spiritual energies which can be transcendent. Yet, nearly everyone is hampered in the search for sexual fulfilment at some point, whether it is by loss of desire, or low libido, which can strike anyone at any time, or outright sexual dysfunction, perhaps involving an underlying health condition, when a person just can't perform under any circumstances no matter how hard he – or she – tries. Although a lot of publicity has been given to male loss of desire and sexual dysfunction, both can – and do – affect women. This book is addressed to both sexes, as well as to partners of people who seem to be suffering from lack of sexual interest.

INTRODUCTION

When you make love is it an overwhelming and rejuvenating experience, or does it just seem like one big unrewarding effort? Is your love life 'all right', but lacking fire? Do you find it easier just to turn over and go to sleep than try yet again to arouse a partner who just doesn't seem interested any more? If you are one of the many people who put up with a less than satisfactory sex life, the chances are that you feel sad, angry and frustrated. Perhaps you are beginning to doubt your own attractiveness and wondering what happened to all that sexual potential you used to be so sure you had.

The message of this book is: don't give up. Too often, people go through life with their sexuality on hold just because they are not aware how easily difficulties such as low libido and sexual dysfunction can be resolved. You may have read a lot about Viagra, for example, but feel it's not for you, or you may decide that you don't want to take a drug for what should be a natural process. Drugs have side-effects, especially if used incorrectly. And if not Viagra, what else is there? Men can choose from a handful of awkward devices for the penis, women may be given antidepressants, and both men and women can have counselling. The options are limited, even crude.

But these sometimes crushing sexual problems can be treated by simple, natural means which are within everyone's reach, and which don't resort to drugs or unsatisfactory medical devices. You can have your sexuality back – and in ways which will leave you feeling generally energized, too. This book is about regaining that sexuality within the context of better all-round health. A healthy sexuality reflects a healthy body, mind and spirit. If you are in search of lost desire, a holistic approach is often far more effective than going to the doctor and getting medical treatments which may treat the sexual organs but not the sexual being, or impotence drugs which go to the other extreme in that they may affect not just one part of the body but the whole of the body.

Many highly effective natural therapies exist to help boost libido. This book looks in some detail at natural aphrodisiacs and dietary supplements which can help restore flagging sexuality. Nature has provided a wealth of herbs and other substances which have been used around the world for centuries as a natural way to boost sexual potency. Some have been well-kept secrets; others are only now being discovered. Yet others have a long-established folk pedigree which is now being substantiated by scientific experiments. You may not be able to visit the mountains of China the Brazilian rainforest to sample the therapies in their place of origin, but it may well be that working your way through them provides a memorable journey of another kind. Combined with other lifestyle factors, such as diet, exercise and rest, natural remedies can not only be very effective in luring back lost desire, but can also dramatically improve your general health and wellbeing.

Sex is closely linked with health, and sexual problems often go much further than being deprived of sex. Physically, they may be part of a package of other minor complaints – lack of energy, headaches, tummy complaints – which you wouldn't visit the doctor about, but which undermine you on a day-to-day basis. Tackling lifestyle issues which underlie sexual difficulties may lead to the resolution of other long-standing difficulties, too.

Many people today are questing for treatments which fill more needs than can be met by the doctor. This book also looks at alternative treatments and therapies, which work on an emotional and spiritual level as well as a physical one, an area where today you are spoilt for choice. Alternative treatments can directly help enhance sexuality, and help eliminate the stress and anxiety which can ruin relaxed physical intimacy. Many of the so-called New Age therapies – often not new at all but the heritage of ancient cultures – can powerfully enhance your general energy, health and wellbeing. These remedies are especially good if you want more out of life in general, for example if you feel that sexual boredom reflects general boredom. Alternative treatments can improve –

even transform – many other areas of your life, making you sharper in mind, freer in spirit and more ready to enjoy the creative and humorous side of life.

Finally, it helps to keep it all in perspective. Building in room for a few disappointments and keeping expectations realistic may help take the tension out of the whole business. It can take time to work miracles but, if you're willing to try, they can happen. You are in control of your sexuality to a far greater extent than you might think, and the way forward can be very simple. And by following the measures suggested in this book you are also building up a solid future in terms of your physical, emotional and spiritual health – and hopefully having fun along the way.

CHAPTER ONE

Why Natural Aphrodisiacs?

SEX is like food – almost anything will do to satisfy appetite and keep the species alive. But getting what you really want can be another matter. Through diffidence, fear or physical problems, too many people hold back when sharing themselves with their partner, so missing out on enjoyment. There are also those for whom lovemaking has become a habit in which nothing is unexpected, who perhaps feel that life is passing them by, or that they are capable of more. Then there are the unwilling sufferers – people whose partners don't seem to want them any more; or, perhaps most frustrating, those who are willing but not able.

Psychologically and emotionally, the costs of lost sexuality can be enormous. A few unsatisfactory encounters can dent confidence for a long time. Men commonly retreat from trying to make love after a few erectile failures, leaving their partner wondering if they're ill or have found someone else. Women who are always too tired to make love, or keep missing out on orgasm, may also withdraw from a situation or even a relationship which no longer seems to have anything to offer but hard work and frustration. Couples often engage in a kind of tacit avoidance of each other, so denying themselves not just sex but closeness and touch in general. So begins the process of silently drifting apart; or taking out the anger and hurt on your partner, so generating more distance; or blaming yourself. Sex is such a sensitive issue that it is all too easy to write yourself off as a failure, or to believe that your problem is unique and impossible to cure. Loss of desire takes many different forms and has many degrees, but the results are similar – disappointment, sadness, anger and loneliness.

For some people, the quality of their sex life is not an issue. They may have other priorities, or be too busy, or be content with occasional, good-enough sex with an established, long-term partner. However, even then there may be special occasions when they might want to spice things up! And, for those who feel the nag of ongoing dissatisfaction, or hear the inner whisper that things could be better, it is very different. Then, lack of intimacy and warmth can result in sterility, anger or other negative emotions. While no one can demand sexual satisfaction as a right, people's feelings when deprived can be very elementary, grounded as they are in core needs. Feeling rejected sexually, it can be all too easy to feel rejected and unloved as a person, or just write off a huge portion of your life on the grounds that 'I'm not really a sexual person'. It doesn't have to be like that. Parts of yourself that appear dead can be brought back to life again. This book will explain how.

Where do natural aphrodisiacs come in?

Classically, the phallus has always been regarded as a kind of buffoon god in the shape of Priapus, god of fertility. The fact that much Greek art shows his elephantine phallus to be the same size and weight as the rest of his body illustrates the attitude to sex we've inherited today – as something which somehow exists apart from the rest of our lives.

More recently, the Viagra phenomenon shows we still hold this view. We all long for a pill to solve the thornier problems of intimacy!

But, though it sometimes seems like it, sex doesn't really have a life of its own. It reflects your general health, wellbeing, lifestyle and relationships. Sometimes poor sex can be a reliable barometer of when things are going wrong physically; sometimes it reflects conflicts within a partnership; sometimes it is a direct response to life stresses such as a leaking roof, no money or a new baby. Then there are the 'live-in lodgers' (certainly not lovers!) so many of us are familiar with – those constant feelings of being under the weather, lacking energy, or the constant minor complaints such as headaches, constipation, colds and so on. You might not think of connecting these with loss of desire, but the body works as a whole, and lifestyle factors which affect some parts of the body, such as the digestive system, will also affect the sexual organs. For example, an overdose of whisky doesn't do your stomach or your sex drive any good. Again, you surely know that nicotine is bad for you, but did you know that smoking also has a specific dampening physiological effect on the sex organs? Or that other drugs can do this too, and that poor sexual performance can sometimes be a side-effect of prescribed medication? Or that poor diet can sometimes wipe out your sex drive? (This applies to obesity as well as nutritional deficiencies.) Were you aware that that surge of irritability when your partner asks for sex could perhaps be a low blood sugar reaction caused by faulty eating habits, or because of exhaustion from stress, overwork or lack of sleep? Lifestyle factors are often the most important factors which affect not just your libido but your general level of energy and wellbeing. By focusing on lifestyle issues, you will probably find that not only does your libido improve, but that other things will get better too.

The supplements described in Chapter 2 can play a major part in improving sex drive and many of them will enhance other aspects of your health and wellbeing as well. The African bark extract yohimbe is perhaps the best-known of all natural aphrodisiacs. Interestingly, it seems to have the same ultimate effect as Viagra, in that it is said to improve blood flow to the penis, although using a different mechanism. Yohimbe may also be used, on its own or in combination with other supplements, to give a general boost to the system. Like other natural approaches, sexual enhancers often go beyond sexuality, energizing your body and so in turn energizing your mind and spirit. And, there are plenty to choose from, depending on what you feel you require.

Complementary therapies, as described in Chapter 4, are another option. You might want to explore a remedy such as massage, which is especially apt for men with sexual dysfunction, as good circulation is key to getting and maintaining an erection. Massage also relaxes both men and women and helps them get in touch with and release the tensions and negative emotions which can stifle sexual expression. There are certain key areas which can be massaged, not with the aim of stimulating the so-called erogenous zones, but to encourage blood flow, to relax or to energize. If you feel worn-out, used-up and generally un-sexy, then an internal cleansing treatment, such as detox, which rids the body of many toxins, leaving you wonderfully revitalized may be appropriate. At an emotional rather than a physical level, various therapies exist to help you release and deal with emotions without words, such as art or sound therapy – very apt as sex is the leading language without words. Or, you may feel the need to look for deeper answers to sexual and personal questions which have been troubling you, and a number of paths exist for such seekers, from the ancient art of numerology, the science of numbers, to modern-day sciences such as Human Design, a unique in-depth computer personality analysis which can analyse your relationships and help you get in touch with hidden aspects of yourself. Any of these therapies can help you come to terms with and creatively explore your sexuality, as well as opening perhaps undreamed-of spiritual paths.

It is within this overall structure that the concept of a natural approach comes in. The sex organs are just that – organs like any others in the body, indelibly linked with the emotions and spirit. They need nourishing in the same way as the body needs nourishing – within the context of an emotionally and mentally satisfying life. Sex cannot be regarded in isolation. Natural alternatives can boost the whole body, and may also work on the mind and spirit to create a much more holistic concept of sexual activity.

Why conventional treatments may not be enough

While conventional treatments for sexual dysfunction do have their place, and can be highly effective for many, they are limited. For a start, they are nearly all for men with erectile problems, There is very little treatment available for women beyond antidepressants, counselling or, occasionally, hormonal treatment. Two of these options involve taking drugs, which some people do not want to do, while counselling, useful though it can be in clearing away emotional and psychological debris, may not be appropriate as it won't tackle physical problems. For both men and women there are much simpler measures that can help. For example, the man whose problems are caused by a zinc deficiency (see page 66) will get his potency back far quicker via a zinc supplement from the local health food store than by sitting in the therapist's chair for an hour a week!

Treatments for men certainly have their limitations. The three major treatments for erectile difficulties – vacuum devices, injection therapy and surgical implants – all have drawbacks. To have to fit a device round the penis every time you want an erection (vacuum therapy), or to inject a drug into the penis (injection therapy), militate against spontaneity to say the least. These options frequently involve discomfort, bruising and pain. Injection therapy may also involve complications and side-effects, such as the possibility of fibrosis or scar tissue in the penis owing to repeated injections. The most serious potential side-effect is priapism, or prolonged erection – a medical emergency which, if untreated, can destroy the ability to have an erection for good (see page 29). Surgery, the other option, can implant plastic rods within the penis to induce stiffening – an effect which is permanent. While handy in terms of instant erection on demand, this sometimes isn't as firm as a natural erection, and may have complications in terms of infection or failure of the implant. Perhaps most importantly in terms of this book, all three devices only work on the penis. They certainly won't tackle low energy, nutritional deficiencies, lack of fitness or any of the other myriad factors which can affect the whole body and result in lowered sexual drive.

Viagra, the 'blue pill' which thoroughly caught the public imagination as the aphrodisiac of all time, is alas no cure-all. While it can obtain impressive results, with clinical trial success rates of 65–88 per cent, Viagra is not actually an aphrodisiac, and does not increase libido. It will not even work for a lot of people. Designed for men with erectile dysfunction, it is not effective in the absence of sexual stimulation.

Owing to well-publicized reports of fatalities in connection with this drug, Viagra also has a slightly dented safety image, and, recently re-labelled to meet FDA regulations, now bristles with provisos as to who can and cannot take it: certainly not those already taking nitrates, where the combination can lower blood pressure to a dangerous level. Caution is also advised with several other groups, including those who have or have had a severe heart or liver problem, recent stroke, heart attack or high or low blood pressure. It is not proven that any deaths were directly due to taking Viagra, and Viagra's manufacturers Pfizer say that the drug is safe when used correctly, but this does put quite a lot of onus on your family doctor when prescribing – it's certainly now recommended that physicians check their patients' cardiovascular health before prescribing Viagra. Above all, you may just not want to take a drug which does have acknowledged side-effects such as headaches, flushing, indigestion, dizziness, stuffy nose, blackouts, and temporary vision problems, including 'blue vision' – a blue or green halo.

Viagra belongs to a group of medicines known as phosphodiesterase type 5 inhibitors, which cause blood vessels to dilate or expand. It was originally developed as a treatment for angina, a heart condition usually caused by narrowed arteries. However, during clinical trials, it was realized that the drug increased blood flow to the male genitals and so caused erection even in those previously diagnosed as sexually dysfunctional.

Some of the natural supplements covered in this book are supposed to have a similar effect, such as yohimbe, also said to improve blood flow to the genital area, but with far fewer side-effects. Other natural remedies such as yoga and massage can also improve circulation. For example, Ayurvedic massage on the lower abdomen can directly improve blood flow to the genital area. There's also no reason why these kinds of remedies can't be used by women.

Finally, as already explained, impotence and other sexual difficulties may often be caused by factors which Viagra will not directly address, such as medication use and general health and lifestyle, and tackling these factors may be a better starting solution than taking Viagra or rival drugs such as Vasomax (phentolamine, which also works on the blood vessels in the penis, but in a different way to Viagra).

As you can see, the natural approach may take many forms that can often be used in combination. You may have to work a little at improving your general health level! But, as already stated, the rewards will be worth it because the chances are that you will feel generally, not just sexually, revitalized.

SNIFFING VIAGRA

TWO RESEARCHERS from the University of Kentucky say they have come up with a nasal spray that could cut the time it takes for Viagra to work from up to an hour to 5–15 minutes. According to Lewis Dittert, one of the researchers, they developed the spray because they felt that because of the nature of Viagra's use, people would prefer not to wait up to an hour for results. Dittert and his colleague, Anwar Hussein, say the nasal spray brings Viagra in contact with mucous membranes, getting the active ingredient, sildenafil, into the bloodstream more quickly. At the time of writing, they are waiting for an official comment on this mode of action from Pfizer.

Before you proceed

There are three provisos. One is that you should on no account feel under pressure to achieve some magical, remote goal. Do as much or as little as you like, and remember to count in the small successes. Think of it as an overall process which is ongoing, rather than aimed towards an end. You may find that you see improvements in more areas than you expect.

The second proviso is that, as already mentioned, loss of sex drive can be related to other underlying disorders. These can vary from serious heart trouble or diabetes to simple fatigue caused by overwork or a series of broken nights with a new baby. Severe psychological problems are another issue altogether, though they are probably less common than generally thought as regards sex. Too many people blame themselves and suspect that 'there must be something really wrong with me' if they can't enjoy sex. Don't be too quick to blame mental problems for any sexual difficulties. See your family doctor first, and ensure that there are no major underlying conditions which could be spoiling your love-life.

The third and final proviso relates to your partner. If you don't love your partner, or find him or her sexually alluring, no amount of aphrodisiacs or counselling are going to help. As the ancient Roman writer Seneca said, love is the best magic philtre, 'without potions, without herbs, without any witch's incantation'.

What is a normal sex drive?

In both men and women the sex drive or libido is, like many other bodily functions, affected by a range of hormones. These are under the control of the pituitary gland and of the hypothalamus, which stimulates the release of, among others, the male sex hormone testosterone.

In women the hypothalamus, acting via the pituitary, sends out a stimulating hormone which acts directly on the ovaries. These in turn produce oestrogen and progesterone, two vital hormones implicated in reproduction generally, as well as sex drive. What triggers the hypothalamus into action may be mental or physical – touch, smell, or sight.

Sex drive varies widely from individual to individual, and there is really no such thing as 'normality'. It is important not to take too much notice of surveys which suggest that most 'normal' couples make love two to three times a week, which is the most common findings of such research. This is an average only and may be highly unrealistic for many couples with perfectly normal sexuality. In general, younger couples tend to have more sexual activity, and this tends to lessen after two years of being together. However, even sex therapists have great difficulty in saying what is a normal sex drive because it varies so much.

The two main problems

The two main problems covered in this book deal with the same thing, but in different degrees. They can be classified as follows:

LOSS OF DESIRE OR LOWERED LIBIDO

This could be said to apply to the fluctuations and dips in sex drive from which we may all suffer at times, and applies to both men and women. It's that feeling that you're just too tired, can't be bothered, or are hard to turn on despite your partner's most loving attentions. It may well vanish with a good night's sleep – many working people say they feel like sex in the morning, but not at night when they fall into bed exhausted. Again, if you're under a lot of pressure at work, you may find you can make love at weekends or on holiday, but not during the working week. Most people with loss of libido can manage sex sometimes, if conditions are right or they make an effort. Simple self-help measures can often boost libido. By following the libido-boosting guidelines in this book, it is likely that you will feel more ready for sex and more able to perform.

SEXUAL DYSFUNCTION

This term can be used to refer to more serious, ongoing inability to enjoy sex, and may sometimes mean that there is some underlying disease or disorder which is contributing to loss of interest – diabetes and heart trouble are two common ones, for example. The term sexual dysfunction is usually applied to men, and may also be called male erectile dysfunction, or impotence, which just means the inability to get and maintain an erection. Although the butt of many jokes, impotence, which affects one in ten men, should always be taken seriously and should result in a visit to the doctor. Women are not usually considered to have an equivalent disorder, although with the increased discussion of the subject following the publicity given to Viagra there is new interest in whether a similar condition exists in women, caused by a lack of blood supply to the female erectile tissues.

The old-fashioned, rather pejorative term frigidity – fairly meaningless anyway – is not really used today. But, there's no doubt that there is a great deal of hidden sexual suffering in women, including inorgasmia or inabilty to reach orgasm.

People with sexual dysfunction will probably find that they can rarely have sex even when circumstances are good. The advice given in this book will help with all sorts of health problems and can improve sexual dysfunction even when severe, but you may need medical help as well, whether that's conventional or alternative. If you do want to consult an alternative practitioner, Chapter 4 looks at treatments which may be particularly useful.

Why do people lose interest?

A survey by National Relate, the UK counselling organization, 'Psychosexual Therapy at Relate', by Peter McCarthy and Marj Thoburn, analysed the sexual habits of nearly 3,700 people. The survey found that, while only 7 per cent of men said they experienced loss of desire or interest, this rose to 39 per cent in women – not only a huge gulf between the sexes, but an increase of 50 per cent on previous estimates. One explanation is that women are no longer prepared to put up with sexual dissatisfaction as the previous generation may have been. Also, women very often lose interest due to an inept or insensitive partner. Sheer lack of sexual technique may contribute. Another common problem is said to be different arousal rates – traditionally, men are supposed to become aroused more quickly than women, and are ready for intercourse before women.

But is it really true that women experience more dissatisfation than men? Or do men just class their dissatisfaction differently, perhaps because of organic differences between the sexes? The same survey showed that 41 per cent of the men had problems such as erectile difficulties and premature ejaculation – surely also signs of dissatisfaction.

But, no matter how you define sexual dissatisfaction, if there was one thing which this survey did show clearly, it was that lack of interest and sexual problems have many causes. Relate's research showed that sexual difficulties often reflected existing dissatisfactions within the relationship. Life issues such as money and housing problems also played a part – enjoyable sex can become something of a luxury if you're worrying about finding money for the mortgage. In the rest of this chapter we will look at the many factors which can influence sex drive.

Does vasectomy affect sex drive?

SOME COUPLES find that the man's sex drive increases dramatically after vasectomy. It is thought that this may be because after vasectomy, blood levels of testosterone go up, as testosterone is absorbed back into the body instead of being secreted. However, other research has found that testosterone levels are lower than normal 10 years after the operation, which may in turn cause libido to drop. It could also be that freedom from care as regards causing pregnancy may also have a liberating effect on the sex drive, the thrill of which may also wear off over the years. On the other hand, a few men suffer temporary impotence after a vasectomy, but this is thought to be due to psychological factors, not physical ones.

Causes of lowered sex drive

Probably most people can recall the occasional off-night, for example after a hard day at work, an over-enthusiastic party or the first night with a new partner. Most often, the causes of low libido in both men and women are simple – tiredness, stress, overwork and lifestyle factors such as diet, smoking and drinking alcohol – and are simply tackled. It may only take a holiday and some healthy eating to put you right, and to restore you to all your former energy and more.

Ongoing sexual dysfunction, which doesn't respond to easy self-help measures, and persistent sexual failure may need more investigation.

The most common causes of poor sexual performance, which are all discussed further in the course of this book, relate to *lifestyle, physical causes* and *psychological causes*. Lifestyle issues are most likely to result just in loss of desire in men and women; physical and psychological causes may cause both mild loss of libido and more serious sexual dysfunction.

LIFESTYLE

Lifestyle is one of the most common causes of loss of desire in both men and women. While this doesn't mean an actual health condition (these are discussed in the next section) lifestyle factors may well affect not just libido but your general level of energy and wellbeing, as discussed in the opening of this chapter. Several factors can contribute to this less-than-optimum feeling, either by themselves or in combination.

Sleep and rest

Not getting enough sleep is a surprisingly common reason for loss of desire in both men and women. Sometimes fatigue may have special significance – for example, fatigue after a viral illness or the exhaustion associated with being bereaved – but should gradually pass off. If it does not, you should see your doctor. In general, though, sleep and rest are matters of habit, and it is possible to 'train' yourself to get enough of both.

Stress

Stress is a notorious passion-killer. This may be a question of everyday worries – pressure at work, money worries, housing problems and so on. A very common reason for switching off is a temporary life situation – sometimes, outside events impinge so much that circumstances just aren't right for intimacy, when you need to feel safe and relaxed. For example, life events such as moving house or changing jobs may absorb all your energy for a while, though most people recover naturally once the crisis is over. Another very common example is a new baby, when dirty nappies, sore breasts from feeding, and broken nights mean that for a few weeks or months the last thing you feel like is a burst of passionate lovemaking.

Nutritional factors

Adequate nutrition can play a vital part in libido, and has many ramifications, from everyday healthy eating, to specific nutritional deficiencies and allergies, or the problems caused by obesity.

Smoking, alcohol and recreational drugs

Smoking and alcohol are both major libido-killers – they both reduce libido directly, and also lower general health, so making strong sexual performance even less likely. Some recreational drugs also lower libido.

Fitness

One factor that is sometimes overlooked is ordinary fitness – sex is after all a physical activity which uses muscles and energy like other activities.

Personal hygiene

Lastly, one lifestyle factor we probably all prefer not to have close encounters with is lack of hygiene – bad breath and smelly socks are more common turn-offs than you might think. Fortunately, once one partner has had the courage to point it out to the other, this is something which can usually be easily remedied.

PHYSICAL PROBLEMS

Physical problems connected with low libido and sexual dysfunction can be many and varied. They may affect the whole body, as with a condition such as diabetes, or they may be confined to the reproductive organs.

Underlying disease

In men, impotence is considered to be a serious medical condition by many experts, and one which may be a warning sign of underlying disease. Because of this it is important to report it to your doctor. Diabetes is the most common cause of sexual dysfunction in men, with erectile dysfunction affecting an estimated 50–60 per cent of diabetic men. Impotence may also be an early sign of heart disease and some cancers. Other physical conditions linked with impotence include multiple sclerosis, high blood pressure, kidney disease, hardening of the arteries (atherosclerosis), fibrosis, hormonal imbalances, nerve damage and epilepsy and other neurological problems. The ageing factor also plays its part. More 'local' physical causes also exist, such as venous leak, a condition in which the penis fills with blood as normal, but the blood then drains away through the veins instead of remaining trapped within the penis.

Hormones

Lower levels of testosterone or oestrogen can affect sexual desire in men and women, so it is a good idea to have a check-up for physical causes. Rarely, this may indicate disease of the hypothalamus or pituitary glands which release the sex hormones affecting desire. Problems with the testicles may be implicated in loss of sex drive, especially if it is sudden. Women may notice individual fluctuations associated with their monthly cycle or with major hormonal events – pregnancy, the postnatal period and menopause. Women taking hormonal medication, including the contraceptive pill, may also find their sex drive is affected.

Infection

Infections such as herpes, thrush (candida) or urethritis can all cause irritation or pain in men. Women may be affected by infections such as thrush, trichomoniasis, genital herpes or bacterial infections which can also cause pain, along with other symptoms including changes in vaginal discharge, itching or blisters. Other potential problem areas are in the cervix, uterus, tubes or ovaries, such as pelvic inflammatory disease (an inflammation of the uterus and tubes caused by infection) or fibroids (often benign growths in the uterus). Other symptoms may include heavy, painful or irregular periods, bleeding between periods or after intercourse, low tummy pain or weight loss.

Structural and sensitivity problems

These are far less common than some people suspect, and as with other sexual matters, normality covers a wide range. In women, structural problems may affect the vagina or hymen. For example a naturally small vaginal opening can cause problems but this is easily corrected by surgery. Post-surgery problems may sometimes cause pain. For example, the shape of the vagina can be changed after an operation for incontinence or prolapse. Insufficient lubrication can also cause pain. This can vary from individual to individual, and may also happen at menopause, and may be helped by a use of water-based lubricant. Men are occasionally affected by Peyronie's disease in which a lump of fibrous tissue develops along the penis, causing it to bend so that a full erection cannot be achieved.

Painful sex

Painful sex (dyspareunia) is more common in women than in men – in fact, it's one of the most common reasons why women consult a gynaecologist. As with men, pain should always mean a consultation with the doctor. Women should also have cervical smears regularly, as painful sex can be a result of infection (see above). Occasionally painful sex, with the anxiety it can cause, can contribute to vaginismus, when the vaginal muscles contract so as to make intercourse impossible. Vaginismus is the most common reason why marriages are not consummated and is thought to affect five of every thousand women and forms up to around 40 per cent of the sexual therapist's workload.

Generally, painful sex in men is almost always due to a physical cause. These are manifold and pain should always be checked out by your doctor, as you may need treatment in the form of medication, or referral to a sexual health clinic or urologist. An overactive cremaster muscle which causes the scrotum to contract can result in spasmodic pain during sex, especially in young men. Pain after ejaculating, sometimes extreme, can also sometimes be caused by sensitivity in the glans of the penis. Causes of painful sex in men include trauma such as small tears in the skin of the penis (sometimes caused by over-enthusiastic use!) tight foreskin or allergic skin reactions to rubber or to the lubricant in condoms.

Medication

Many drugs can wipe out desire and performance, including high blood pressure medicines, oral contraceptives, antidepressants and some diuretics and seizure medications. If you notice a sudden change in sexual desire after taking a medication, consult your doctor.

PSYCHOLOGICAL AND EMOTIONAL FACTORS

Once your doctor has excluded physical problems, you may want to consider whether psychological or emotional factors are playing a part in any difficulties. Sometimes a combination of factors may be operating. Deep-rooted emotional, psychological and social issues which affect sexual experience may need addressing separately, and may be beyond the scope of the remedies suggested in this book – though it is certainly worth trying these first. Many people have found that mental and emotional 'problems' magically disappear when they improve their diet or find the right supplement. The mental effects of poor nutrition are well-documented. To take just one example, irritability (and loss of interest in sex) can be a sign of deficiency in several nutrients including B vitamins and manganese (See Chapter 3.)

The other main consideration is your relationship with your partner – how good it is, and, in particular, how good you both are at communication. Research shows that good communication is key in working through any difficulties together. What works is being open about fears and worries, avoiding secrecy and avoiding blame (yourself or your partner); deciding if you're both motivated to resolve the problem; deciding what to do about it (i.e. visiting the doctor, self-help measures, complementary therapies); and keeping a sense of humour – not always easy, but vital for overall as well as sexual health!

Relationship conflicts

One point to consider is whether lack of sex drive is 'global', that is, with all partners and in all situations, or if it only occurs with a certain partner or in certain situations. Low sexual desire can sometimes reflect problems in a relationship. For example, one partner may withhold sex as a way of expressing hostility, or may use intimacy and personal boundaries as a weapon when what really needs to be discussed is money – quite common, according to therapists at National Relate. Sometimes too much damage has been done within the relationship and some people find that the only solution is a change of partner but, on the positive side, the Relate survey mentioned earlier in this chapter also found that many of the couples they surveyed had good responses to psychosexual therapy, with most couples reporting improvements after counselling.

Sexual boredom

First-night nerves with a new partner, or sexual inexperience, can freeze sexual enjoyment. It takes time to establish a good sexual relationship with another person. But at the other end of the scale, creeping boredom can slowly destroy a sexual relationship as time goes by. Many people believe that sex should be totally natural and spontaneous, though sex therapists say that sex is in fact an area which does respond to effort, and that couples can revitalize their sex lives with new strategies. The younger you are, the more often you are likely to make love, but, generally, after two years in a relationship you tend to make love less often, and after five years statistics show that the numbers of times you make love drops each year by an average of one time a month.

Psychological problems

Lack of desire can reflect a fear of intimacy, or be a symptom of depression or more serious personality disorders which make it hard to connect with others and integrate love and sexuality. Some people with low desire have disturbed backgrounds which include memories of trauma such as abuse or rape, and may have difficulty being sexually intimate in a safe, committed relationship. These problems probably need specialist counselling or psychiatric help.

So now what?

You now have a good overview of several possible factors that can affect sex drive, and maybe you want to take action and start working on them right away. But, before tackling the problem yourself, it is advisable to have a medical check-up as suggested earlier on in this chapter to make sure that there is no underlying physical factor which could be implicated in loss of sex drive. By taking a detailed medical history, and arranging blood and other tests, your doctor will be able to help you decide whether sexual problems exist by themselves, or as a part of some other condition. Once you've excluded underlying physical problems, you are free to experiment.

THE CHASTITY OPTION

FACING SEXUAL PROBLEMS doesn't mean that you have to resume sex. Some people find, perhaps to their surprise, that once they've discussed their problems, they are actually quite content with matters as they stand and would prefer not to make efforts to have a sex life. This can be a surprisingly liberating decision for many, though some may go through feelings of guilt or a sense of inadequacy. Chastity was for centuries one of the leading Christian virtues, and sublimated sexual energy is said to be the driving force behind much medieval and Renaissance art and music. It is still prized in some philosophies and religions today as a means of conserving energy for other purposes. Chastity can of course also be temporary and reversible.

CHAPTER TWO

Natural Remedies

SINCE time immemorial people have tried natural remedies which promise to lift libido. Natural remedies were there long before Viagra and they will almost certainly be there for all foreseeable time to come. Today the market is flooded with 'male support herbs', 'sensual buys', 'virility remedies' and the like – a variety of herbs, plant extracts and nutrients all designed to encourage sexual potency, without the side-effects of heavy-duty drugs and often at a fraction of the cost.

Our approach to health is undergoing a radical change, reflected by the fact that the sale of natural products has increased by 200 per cent over the past five years We are becoming more flexible, more willing to experiment and less dependent on conventional medicine. As we move towards the 21st century, we are increasingly resuming responsibility for our own health and wellbeing, and the interest in natural remedies reflects this. This applies particularly to sexual matters, which you may not view as a health problem so much as a personal, private matter. As already stated, it is important to check out sexual dysfunction with your doctor, but if, as is very likely, you are given the all-clear, what then? Being medically fit can be a minimal definition which may not encompass the fullness of energy and joy in living promised by many alternative remedies.

What attracts many people to alternative remedies is their holistic element. The word holistic derives from the Greek 'holos' meaning whole, and as such aims to treat the person as a complete being, aiming to balance and harmonize mind, body and spirit, rather than isolating a disease and treating the symptoms. Holistic healing techniques depend on centuries of learned skills, passed down from practitioner to practitioner. This chapter looks at supplements you can take to boost sexual performance, which are different to conventional medication because they have been used with this holistic concept in mind.

We have inherited a strong tradition in the use of natural aphrodisiacs in the West, especially with regard to herbal remedies, and even though it has largely been forgotten, it is still there, just waiting to be resurrected. Love potions were among the mainstays of the stock of any self-respecting ancient herbalist or apothecary, who might have used an extraordinary range of products, including the claws, inner organs and urine of animals, which may at least have helped distract those desperately in love! Traditionally, there was a strong element of magic mixed in with herbal crafts, although herbalists such as Culpeper, the 17th-century practitioner, did much to establish the purity of the practice and found a tradition which has been handed down to us today.

Disciplines from other cultures also contribute to the wealth of knowledge at out fingertips, such as African tribal traditions, Traditional Chinese Medicine (TCM), and the ancient art of Ayurveda. These days, we are especially privileged in that the wealth of printed matter on offer and our sophisticated communications technology makes it possible to share knowledge in hours or days which in previous centuries it would have taken years to learn.

Last, but by no means least, is the question of availability. A very wide range of supplements and herbs can be found in natural healthcare or specialist herbal stores. People of any age or sex can derive positive benefits from the wealth of these gentle choices on offer today. When it's all so available, why miss out?

The aphrodisiac story

'Aphrodisiacks, Things that excite Lust or Venery', as the 1719 dictionary *Glossographia Anglicana Nova* puts it, are substances which are supposed to increase sexual desire and performance. However, these days they often come perilously near to being treated as jokes as many of them have merely been chosen for their resemblance to genitalia. This reflects a lingering belief in sympathetic magic – a topic much explored in James Frazer's classic history of myth and religion, *The Golden Bough*. According to sympathetic magic, an object which resembles another object can affect it, so foods which look like an erect penis (banana or asparagus, for example) are said to have a direct action on these organs, and to act as male stimulants. Likewise, enclosed foods such as the oyster are thought to help women. The most infamous aspect of aphrodisiacs is the hunting of animals for some particular supposedly aphrodisiac part, such as rhinoceros horn, whose only value is its phallic shape.

Named after Aphrodite, Greek goddess of love, many aphrodisiacs have a long folk history, but only in selected cases do they actually seem to be effective, though of course the psychological effects of eating something you believe will work can't be ignored. In some cases, aphrodisiacs seem to act as a general stimulant – for example, chocolate contains the stimulant theobromine (see page 26). In other cases, there may be a nutritional basis. For example oysters, renowned for their aphrodisiac qualities, contain a lot of zinc, a mineral necessary for male fertility and optimal testosterone levels, and which is lost in large amounts via semen. Casanova was reputed to eat 50 a day! Oysters and other seafood may also have gained their reputation from Aphrodite's connection with the sea – she is said to have risen naked from the sea on a scallop shell, near Paphos, in Cyprus. Other noted aphrodisiacs include spicy foods, vanilla bean, liquorice root, onions, peaches, blackcurrants, blackberries, leeks, broccoli, parsnips, spinach and tomatoes. Perhaps in times gone by, when the fresh produce could only be had in season, people were so low in the vitamins and minerals they offered that their consumption provided a terrific burst of nutrients which effectively did the trick.

SOME TRADITIONAL APHRODISIACS

Many different substances have starred as aphrodisiacs over the centuries: asses' milk was favoured by the Romans, for example, and monkey urine by the Kama Sutra – both it would seem for external rather than internal use.The following are some of the best known.

Chocolate

When Cortes plundered Mexico and the Aztec kingdom of Montezuma in 1519, part of his booty was a certain 'food of the gods' claimed to have potent aphrodisiac qualities. Montezuma is reported to have consumed 50 cups of chocolate a day to help sustain his activities in the harem. *Chocolatl* consisted of raw cacao beans (*Theobroma cacao*), red peppers and various herbs, and was reputedly rather bitter. In 1550 nuns in Chiapas followed this up with another, also supposedly aphrodisiac, and more palatable cocoa brew, with cacao beans, vanilla and sugar. The active ingredient theobromine is the main stimulant though hot red peppers doubtless added something to its kick.

More recently Dr Michael Liebowitz of the New York State Psychiatric Institute did a study showing that the phenylethylamine (PEA) in chocolate releases the same feel-good hormones that flow during lovemaking. Actually cheese contains around 10 times more PEA than chocolate, and cheese is considered an aphrodisiac in Italy. Other foods with a high PEA content are almonds, apples, avocados, peanuts, pineapple, tomatoes, chicken, beef and spinach.

Tobacco

Much of the early success of tobacco was due to its supposedly aphrodisiac qualities. Its potency was taken seriously in some countries – in China, Japan and Persia smoking was prohibited and those caught having a puff were executed. Tobacco is sacred to the Natives of America and is believed to have supernatural powers to harm and heal as well as to create affection between man and woman. The word tobacco is an adaptation from an Arawak term (Columbus discovered tobacco among the Arawaks of the West Indies). In Native North American mythology and ritual, tobacco is offered to the Great Spirit, the spirits of the wind, moon, sun, water and thunder. The smoke, which embodies the breath, carries prayers and messages. Tribes of South America, the Pacific, the Caribbean and elsewhere use tobacco in shamanic and other rituals. The pleasure of smoking has a proven physiological basis as it is known to be caused by the active ingredient nicotine, which interacts with nicotinic receptors in the brain to cause the pleasurable 'charge' of smoking.

Nutmeg

Nutmeg became renowned as an aphrodisiac (and also as a soporific and abortifacient) after the Portuguese discovered the tree *Myristica fragrans* on the Banda Islands off Indonesia in 1512. In the 1970s, prisoners in US jails experimented with hot milk and powdered nutmeg but the resulting 'high' was usually outweighed by the hangover which followed. It isn't actually known why nutmeg is intoxicating.

Alcohol

Alcohol was renowned as an aphrodisiac in Ancient Greece, where wine drinking was well-established, and has retained its reputation to this day, though usually with the equally notorious effect of improving desire but impairing performance. In particular, absinthe, 'La Fée Verte', the Green Fairy, which came into being in the 1700s, was notorious for producing sometimes wild sexual excitement and stimulating the mind. However, it also produced terrifying hallucinations and eventually a condition known as 'absinthism', when drinkers became weakened in body and mind and usually died early, often by suicide.

A 1994 study published in the journal *Nature* suggests there may be more to alcohol's role. According to the study, alcohol raises women's levels of testosterone, a hormone linked to libido in both sexes.

Honey

Honey has been viewed as an aphrodisiac throughout history. Newly weds in ancient Europe mixed it with wine to boost their stamina (hence the term 'honeymoon', a month of honey). The ancient Arabs went in for topical application. The classic erotic text *The Perfumed Garden* recommends honey and ginger rubbed on the penis as a

Priapism and Priapus

PRIAPISM, mentioned above (see page 6 and also Spanish fly page 30) is prolonged erection, or when erection lasts for more than four hours. It is also a medical emergency, which, if left untreated, can permanently destroy the ability to have an erection. After a normal erection blood usually naturally drains away from the penis back into the body via the corpora cavernosum (known as detumescence). Priapism is when this does not occur, and it is dangerous because of the risk of blood clotting in the corpora cavernosa. This kind of thrombosis produces senous and long-term damage. Priapism needs urgent treatment, which may include letting some of the trapped blood out with a wide-bore needle.

The condition, as is obvious, gets its name from the rather happier Priapus, the Greek fertility god of orchards and gardens with an immense sense of humour and equally large phallus, who guarded the produce by threatening scrumpers with impalement on his elephantine organ. In ancient Greek times, the size of the phallus formed a language of its own in statues and works of art – big ones seem to have been linked with obscenity, buffoonery, lust, luck and fertility; droopy ones indicated senility; and circumcized ones, self-control. They were a potent symbol for women also, and figured in a number of women-only festivals in the form of phallic costumes and phallic cakes.

'prescription for increasing the dimensions of small members and for making them splendid'.

Potatoes

When first introduced into Europe in the 16th century, potatoes were only popular as aphrodisiacs. They sold for as much as £250 a pound – at that time, it would have taken the average labourer 20 years to earn that sum.

Spanish Fly

Spanish fly has a well-established aphrodisiac reputation, just as strongly countered by a long line of exasperated doctors pronouncing its reputation to be totally undeserved. Also known as cantharides and made from dried blister beetles, *Cantharis vesicatoria*, it may be effective because it irritates the urethra. It can also cause priapism in men as well as prolonged stimulation of the female erectile tissue, and may be

Bread of Love

APHRODISIACS could take strange and active forms which approximated to a magic ritual. Burchard I, Bishop of Worms 100–125, describes how one method of raising desire was linked with the harvest, and possibly has echoes of old European fertility rites. When the wheat had been harvested, a woman who desired a particular man would undress and roll around over it. The wheat was then threshed and taken to the mill and the flour used to prepare love breads', which were supposed to cause immediate desire for the woman when she gave them to the man of her choice.

dangerous because of the risk of blood clotting or thrombosis because the blood can't drain out (see box Priapism and Priapus).

A history of pharmacy – the origins of herbal medicine

The medicinal effects of plants was discovered by the ancients and the word pharmacy is derived from the Greek *pharmakon*, drug. The idea that the gods taught humans herbal medicine was prevalent in ancient times.*The Book of Enoch*, an ancient Ethiopian text written between the first and second centuries BC, describes how angels married human women and taught them how to make medicines out of plants – a story which effectively links sexual union and medicinal power. In making women the first herbalists, this story also foreshadows later developments in which some of the greatest herbalists have been women. It also echoes several biblical references to herbal medicine, such as Ecclesiasticus 38:4, 'The Lord hath created medicines out of the earth.'

The earliest systematic study of herbal medicine was made by the Emperor Shennung (or Shen Nong), thought to have lived around 2700BC. Supposed to have poisoned himself 80 times a day, he always found an antidote because of his superlative knowledge of herbs. The *Shennung Herbal* mentions the medicinal uses of 356 drugs.

The ancient Egyptians also made extensive and often colourful use of natural products – one remedy designed to allure the opposite sex, for Queen Shesh of Egypt, included claw of dog, decayed palm leaves and the hoof of an ass! The Ebers Papyrus written in 1500BC, lists over 800 remedies.

Greeks and Romans documented the many herbs they used.

Theophrastus (370–285BC) made a classification of plants *Historia Plantarum* and Pliny was just one of the Roman writers who wrote widely about medicinal plants. The Greek doctor Galen (around AD129 –199) also worked as a herbalist.

In the Dark Ages in Europe, the knowledge of herbal remedies was mainly passed on in 'leechbooks' (from the Anglo-Saxon, *laece*, to heal) which were mainly superstitious remedies against evil forces such as goblins. From around the 10th century, the monks became renowned as masters of herbal lore, details of which were kept in their extensive libraries. (Interestingly, to this day it is said that only two monks at any one time from La Grande Chartreuse, near Grenoble, France, are ever allowed to know the secret herbal ingredients of the famous liqueur, once said to have love-enhancing properties.)

Nicholas Culpeper (1616–1654) was the great figure of British herbalism. Culpeper's own love-life received a bizarre and abrupt termination when the heiress he was eloping with was killed as lightning struck her coach. Culpeper, traumatized it would seem by the event, abandoned his studies at Cambridge and became an apothecary, causing much ill-will among the medical establishment by treating the poor for free and translating the Latin pharmacopoeia into English so that everyone could understand it. In those times, only an educated handful knew Latin, and before Culpeper herbal knowledge was a jealously guarded secret, available only to medics. Culpeper sought to make this knowledge widely available and his works, including his *Herbal*, were very popular during his lifetime, widely used until the 19th century, and are still read today. Culpeper suggests asparagus, mint, mustard seed and onion among others 'to provoke lust' – though he thought that lettuce works against the sexual urge and cucumbers, despite their phallic appearance, also dampen down desire because they are cold and moist.

In the late 19th century a number of small companies set up specializing in the production of plant extracts and were the forerunners of the modern pharmaceutical company – although in fact drug discovery based on naturally occurring herbs and other substances did not begin until well into the 20th century.

Around 80 per cent of drugs today have their basis in natural sources such as plants, and pharmaceutical companies are actively exploring – some would say exploiting – native sources of botanical wisdom, such as the Amazonian Indians. This traditional native knowledge has its roots in the main evidence for the efficacy of natural remedies – centuries of what could be called working proof, handed down by word of mouth, knowledge unlikely to be wasted in traditional rural areas where self-reliance is key, and where shopping around from therapy to therapy just isn't possible. Knowledge of which herb works, and in what amounts, forms an arcane, highly specialized medical lore which is passed on from healer to healer through several generations. Most pharmaceutical drugs, by contrast, are relatively new – and in fact, it is only this century that pharmaceutical companies have begun to create products which mimic natural resources, a move which has become ever more sophisticated in recent years with the latest computer technology.

HERBS AND SEX

Sex being the melange of physical and emotional factors that it is, herbal remedies will be more effective if the spirit as well as the body is willing. However, given that the frame of mind is right, there are certain herbs that have not got their reputation for nothing. And, as herbal remedies usually work holistically, that is as an

WITCH-DOCTORS AND THE DRUGS COMPANIES

IN SOUTH AFRICA, if you fall in love and want it reciprocated, or find yourself willing but unable to reciprocate someone else's love, you visit a witch-doctor. The ***sangomsa*** are the female traditional healers, and the ***inyangas*** are the male ones. Their remedies are said to be effective. Indeed, if you want proof that natural remedies work, you have only to look at how they are being explored by the pharmaceutical companies, which have a keen nose for profit in one of the most competitive of all industries, and are unlikely to waste time on ineffective folk remedies.

For the Traditional Medical Practitioners and African National Healers Association, 'bio-prospecting' has long been a fact of life, but many traditional healers feel they are not getting recognition and recompense for the exploitation of their knowledge. According to foreign correspondent Sam Kiley in South Africa, writing in the UK's ***Sunday Times*** magazine, there are around 300,000 traditional healers in South Africa, and 80 per cent of South Africans visit them as first choice in preference to Western doctors. Traditional healers root their authority in centuries of proven knowledge, and are more than equipped to treat disorders such as impotence. For example, ***vuku-vuku*** is a herbal mix including parts of a beetle similar to 'Spanish fly' which must be taken in tiny amounts to avoid priapism, or prolonged erection.

But many traditional healers are concerned about the arrival of the pharmaceutical giants, wondering how long it will be before their long-cherished remedies are put through the drug development mill and end up on the shelves of Western pharmacies – expensive, and making millions for the companies, but bringing no profit to their originators. There's also the dubious question of isolating a single ingredient from the complex and subtle blend that makes up traditional medicine. However, the encouraging news is that there are signs of some recognition for the traditional healers, in that some companies are now signing deals with them, rather than simply finding out what they know, and going away to turn the knowledge into profits.

overall stimulant, tonic or re-balancer for the body, you may find yourself pepped up generally as well as sexually. There's no doubt that some herbs do have natural stimulant properties, and the right herb in the right amount can work better than drugs and without their side effects. It may take a little trial and error to discover what works best for you, perhaps trying different products or a combination of products or a different dose. If you prefer, you could get expert advice from a herbalist. However, experimentation is part of the fun – and the fun element shouldn't be overlooked. Giving yourself permission to experiment can be surprisingly effective. As has often been said, the best aphrodisiac is the one which is six inches from lobe to lobe – the human brain.

GETTING IT RIGHT

THE RIGHT DOSE can be essential for success and an incorrect dose can be dangerous, so do follow the dosages recommended by the manufacturers or suppliers. It may also be useful to consult a properly qualified herbalist (see page 55). Some products may need to be treated with caution or avoided altogether by certain people, such as women who are pregnant or breastfeeding, or those with heart trouble or other conditions. It is not always recognized that herbs can clash with conventional medicines, so if you are already taking medication, you are advised to check with your usual doctor that your current medication is compatible with the herb of your choice.

You should also make sure you get your supply from a reliable herbalist or stockist. According to six separate reports published in the ***New England Journal of Medicine***, occasionally impotence can actually be a result of toxic substances or drugs unwlttingly mixed into the products labelled 'all-natural'.

Natural remedies

In the West we are very used to the idea of the single chemical – one fix, one pill, working on a single disorder; it is a well-entrenched part of our view of medicine. But, it is being increasingly recognized that this sometimes aggressive approach to health problems is not always as efficient or effective as we may wish, and can even lead to problems – one in ten hospital admissions are as a result of adverse drug reactions and side-effects. Natural, healthy alternatives, many of them used for thousands of years, are becoming increasingly popular as the balance swings back from high-tech healthcare to more traditional, tried and trusted methods.

Natural alternatives also have a vast benefit in that they treat what might be called sub-optimum health – the things you wouldn't bother the doctor about, and many sexual difficulties fall into this category, particularly lack of sexual energy and low libido. There isn't much on the drug shelf for this. Even Viagra is not designed to boost sex drive.

Paradoxically perhaps, herbalism and the use of other natural remedies underlies much modern drug creation today. Pharmaceutical companies isolate and often synthesize the active ingredient. But many natural-health practitioners believe that this isolation of a single ingredient throws the entire therapeutic effect out of balance, producing powerful often toxic drugs with many side-effects, while natural remedies with their complex mix of ingredients offer a gentler and safer way, allowing the body to re-balance and heal itself without having 'cures' thrust upon it.

Many natural herbs work best if you also adopt a generally healthy lifestyle. For maximum effectiveness, it's worth paying attention to diet and exercise, and making sure you drink in moderation and cut out smoking. Many herbs are slow-acting with a long-term, cumulative effect – so be patient! Because they are gentle and natural, too, the effects may be gradual rather than sudden – it is not like taking a pill an hour before intercourse and waiting for the desired effect!

Natural remedies work in various ways. Some are said to have specific effects on blood flow or other biological mechanisms which increase sexual ability. Some work on the whole body and have an indirect beneficial effect on sexual health; others are adaptogens, meaning they balance the entire system. Whichever remedy you choose, you'll probably find that it has other beneficial effects, too, improving your health and overall quality of life.

The herbs described are mostly available in health stores and specialist herb stores, or by mail order.

YOHIMBE

Yohimbe is widely viewed as the world's leading effective natural aphrodisiac. Yohimbe is the bark from the African tree *Corynanthe yohimbe*, or *Pausinystalis yohimbe,* which grows throughout the African countries of Cameroon, Gabon and Zaire. Folklore says that it was given to young men and women making love for the first time to combat beginners' nerves. In Africa it is still used as a tonic during fertility rituals and today in the West is viewed as a sexual stimulant for men and women. Before the introduction of Viagra, doctors in the US prescribed the drug Yohimbe Hydrochloride (a chemical extracted from the bark of yohimbe) as the only approved Food and Drug Administration (FDA) drug to treat impotence.

Yohimbe bark contains yohimbine, an alkaloid which is said to help stimulate the spinal nerves and increase the blood supply to the pelvic area and the erectile tissues, as well as enhancing the reflexes involved in control of ejaculation. Classified as an 'alpha-2 adrenergic blocking agent', the alkaloid in yohimbe is supposed to reduce the effects of hormones which cause constriction of blood vessels and so may be able to help sexual dysfunction. In particular, yohimbe boosts blood flow to the corpus cavernosum to help engorge the penis. At the same time, yohimbe increases the body's production of norepinephrine, known to be essential to erections, and is also said to boost the supply of the hormone adrenalin to nerve endings, which can increase sensual stimulation.

Yohimbe is also said to also suppress the action of 'ageing hormones'. As an alpha-adrenoreceptor blocker, yohimbe reduces the effect of hormones that cause constriction of blood vessels, which often increases with ageing. Together with lifestyle and dietary changes, yohimbe may be a key to the successful treatment of impotence without drugs. Yohimbe may also help normally functioning men who occasionally want to boost their potency. And, it is also recommended for women.

Yohimbe has undergone clinical trials which have been documented in the *New England Journal of Medicine*. Double blind trials at Stanford University show that yohimbe can increase blood flow to the penis. A clinical study in Rhode Island, published in the *Journal of Urology*, tested the active ingredient in yohimbe on a group of men who had experienced chronic sexual dysfunction. For those who had been impotent for less than two years, the improvement rate was 81 per cent after taking a moderate dose for one month. Two out of three patients who previously had experienced only partial erections, and had failed in normal intercourse at least 50 per cent of the time, now reported fuller and more lasting erections.

Earlier medical studies reported 70–85 per cent improvement rates with impotent patients. A landmark Canadian study in the 1980s showed that the active ingredient in yohimbe could be a significant aid to restoring potency in diabetic and heart patients who often are prey to impotence. Overall the study's success rate for serious organic cases was 44 per cent – startling enough to be prominently reported in *Science Digest*, *Time*, and *Health* magazines as an alternative to invasive treatments.

In a 1994 Italian clinical study, half the patients received the active ingredient for eight weeks and half received placebos. The yohimbe group showed a 71 per cent positive recovery rate, compared to the placebo group's 22 per cent. When the placebo group was changed to yohimbe, it scored a 74 per cent success rate.

Apparently, yohimbe bark does not have the well-known Viagra side-effects such as throbbing headaches, blurred vision, blue or green haloes or blackouts. However, yohimbe does have some have reported side-effects, including anxiety, panic attacks, hallucination, rise in blood pressure and heart rate, dizziness, headache and skin flushing. Side-effects can be warded off by taking a low dose; and some manufacturers have formulated yohimbe in liquid form with a balance of nutrients to aim for maximum absorption by the body and greater effectiveness at a low dosage.

How to take it:

As a tea. Preparations are available from specialist healthcare, healthfood or herbal stores; follow the instructions on the packet.

Caution: yohimbe should not be taken if you have high blood pressure, and you should consult your doctor before taking it if you have any type of heart condition.

Many other products exist apart from yohimbe and these are listed in alphabetical order.

Understanding Sexual Arousal and Blood Flow

A GOOD HEALTHY BLOOD FLOW is vital to effective erection – and is vital for keeping your heart in good working order and preventing conditions such as arteriosclerosis, or furring up of the arteries. In other words, keeping yourself in peak health is key to good blood flow, which is key to good sex! Interestingly, the same applies to women – a good blood flow is what causes clitoral and vulval engorgment, and this swelling, together with increased lubrication, prepares these areas for easy entry of the penis. The clitoris has the same basic structure as the penis in that it is made up of three tubes and also undergoes erection, becoming swollen and stiff with extra blood on arousal.

Blood flow in and out of the penis – and, experts suspect, the clitoral area – can become obstructed if the tiny veins which allow blood in and out get blocked up, just as they can do in the rest of the body. The penis is made up of inflatable erectile tissue, the corpora cavernosum and corpus sponglosum. What happens in an erection is that blood rushes into the penis and fills these tissues so that veins are compressed, trapping the blood so it cannot flow back out again. The erection process can be divided into several stages:

PHASE 0 – the normal flaccid state, with minimal blood flow.

PHASE 1 – the latent or filling phase, with increased blood flow through the pudendal and cavernous arteries.

PHASE 2 – the tumescence phase, when intercavernous pressure increases rapidly and penile engorgement occurs.

PHASE 3 – the full erection phase, when the blood flow stops altogether, with tiny blood vessels compressed by the increased blood volume.

PHASE 4 – Detumescence, when pressure on the tiny blood vessels slackens and blood begins to flow out of the penis, which gradually returns to the normal flaccid state.

Viagra works on an enzyme in the penis which relaxes muscles in the area and dilates or widens blood vessels, so allowing more blood in. Some natural products, like yohimbe, work on boosting blood flow to the penis and genital area, but with a different mode of action to Viagra.

AGNUS CASTUS

Agnus castus berries, or *Vitex agnus-castus*, also known as chaste berry, plays a double role in the sexual game, as it is supposed both to increase sexual desire and damp it down! It fact, agnus castus works by correcting hormonal imbalances, balancing sexual energy in particular, and hopefully leaving you with exactly the right amount of desire and performance! Agnus castus is still used in monasteries to help monks keep to their vows of chastity, by balancing excess male hormones. The fruit of a pretty, half-hardy Mediterranean shrub, the berries have a pleasant, peppery taste when dried.

How to take it: The best time to take the berries is early in the morning, before breakfast.

Decoction To 1oz/25g of berries add 1 pint/500ml boiling water. Leave to infuse for 10 minutes. Drink one to two cups a day.

Tincture 20–30 drops a day in a little water.

With meals Grind two good pinches or a quarter of a flat teaspoon of berries in a coffee grinder and sprinkle on to meals.

CATUABA

Catuaba is a small, strongly aromatic shrub from the Brazilian rainforests whose bark, stem and leaves have been used by the Tupi Indians, who have praised its wonderful effects in restoring lost desire in songs for generations. A member of the *Erythroxylaceae* family, catuaba is said to strengthen and stimulate the entire nervous system, enhance libido, act as a tonic for the reproductive system and for those suffering from restless sleep and insomnia, and it is also supposed to improve memory. Catuaba is meant to have a cumulative, long-term effect first signalled by erotic dreams, and followed by increased sexual desire. It can be used as a libido booster by men and women.

How to take it: Preparations are available from specialist healthcare, healthfood or herbal stores; follow the instructions on the packet.

CELERY

It is increasingly being recognized that common vegetables we tend to take for granted have all sorts of health-giving properties. Celery stimulates the pituitary gland which is involved in the release of the sexual hormones, and the celery root is said to be aphrodisiac. The seeds are rich in iron and many vitamins, including A, B and C, and so celery could be used to help boost desire which has been flagging because of tiredness or poor diet.

How to take it: Best eaten raw – try it with a garlic aioli (see page 44)

Caution: Do not use during pregnancy as celery causes the uterus to contract.

DAMIANA

Damiana, *Turnera aphrodisiaca*, has an ancient erotic reputation, particularly among the Mexican Indians. It is believed it contains alkaloids which could work on the body to help raise levels of testosterone. In the early 1900s Dr W. H. Meyers, an American doctor, gave damiana an extensive trial in his practice and found that 'in cases of partial impotence and sexual debility, its success is universal'. It is said to act as a stimulant tonic on the reproductive system in both men and women. It also has a particular use for impotence and sterility associated with anxiety, especially in men, and it has also been recommended for inflammation of the prostate (for the importance of the prostate in the sexual system, see Chapter 4).

Damiana is known to stimulate the uro-genital tract slightly and to produce mild, short-lived euphoria. It has also been recommended for use in relieving emotional and psychological issues which can affect sex, such as stress.

As well as being renowned as an aphrodisiac, damiana is also classed as a stimulant, tonic and diuretic. It has been used as a remedy for exhaustion, inflammation of the bladder, inflammation of the testicles, and kidney inflammation. It is also used to treat depression, anxiety, poor digestion with constipation and lack of appetite and cystitis.

How to take it: Damiana is generally drunk as a tea around an hour before a sexual encounter although it is sometimes recommended that you take half a cup of this or one teaspoon of the tincture twice a day. Some experts have suggested that it can work better when combined with other herbs, including wild oats or saw palmetto (see page 53). Use one cup of the combination tea, or one teaspoon of the tincture, twice daily.

Caution: Damiana is safe but quite stimulating. Do not exceed the recommended dose.

GARLIC

By all accounts garlic is a natural wonder substance, and is used for a wide range of purposes. It is said to work as a libido-booster, increasing desire and function for both men and women, though if you're worried that it might drive away any potential partner, the smell of garlic on the breath can be reduced by eating an apple, drinking a little fresh lemon juice or eating fresh parsley afterwards.

The ancient Egyptians and Babylonians ate large quantities of garlic and onion, as did the seafaring Vikings and Phoenicians, who warded off scurvy with the vitamin C garlic contains. It has been suggested that the Talmud's recommendation to 'eat garlic on Friday on account of its salutary action' was because of its aphrodisiac qualities.

In recent times, garlic has undergone clinical trials which show beyond doubt that it is certainly good for the heart as it helps keep blood vessels free of blockages by preventing arteriosclerosis, or furring up of the arteries. (This can also be important in treating sexual dysfunction, when you consider the importance of good blood flow for erections.) Several garlic constituents have been identified, including ajoene and methylallyl trisulphide, which are known to help prevent clot formation.

How to take it: Garlic is supposed be slow acting, so allow around a month before you expect effects. You can take garlic capsules – one recommended dose is up to 10 capsules a day, but otherwise follow the manufacturer's instructions. Or, taking the fresh cloves crushed has been recommended for sexual problems You don't have to chew the naked clove – there are several different ways to eat it.

Aioli Use a pestle and mortar if you have one, or a blender. Crush two cloves of garlic, then mix with the yolk of one free-range egg. Gradually add olive oil, at first drop by drop, then as a steady trickle, beating well until you have a thick, yellow mayonnaise. Eat with fresh vegetables (carrots, cauliflower, radishes and celery – see separate entry on celery) for a delicious healthy snack.

Garlic syrup Peel and chop 6–8 garlic cloves, place in a jar and cover with 8 tablespoons of honey. Allow to stand for several days, then strain the garlic-infused honey and take four teaspoons twice a day.

Garlic juice This is great if you have a juicer. Place three cloves of peeled garlic in a blender and add 4 tablespoons of honey, the juice of two lemons and the juice from 1lb/0.5kg fresh beetroot. Beetroot is a blood-booster and can help sexual dysfunction caused by poor blood flow. For more on the benefits of juiced vegetables, see the section on Detoxing in Chapter 3.

Roasted garlic Garlic bulbs are delicious roasted whole, as a starter or side vegetable.

GINGER

Ginger is viewed as an aphrodisiac in Traditional Chinese Medicine and is also used to treat impotence as well as a string of other conditions. Like garlic, it has many uses and is well worth buying regularly when you go shopping. In particular, ginger is used to improve circulation, and therefore it may help erectile dysfunction due to poor circulation – you can feel for yourself the warmth and slight tingle a cup of ginger tea produces through the whole system.

The spice is made from the rhizome, or enlarged underground stem, of the herbaceous plant *Zingiber officinale*. It is native to India, where the ancient Ayurvedics used it to preserve food, as a digestive aid and as a spiritual and physical cleanser. The Greeks wrapped the root in a piece of bread and ate it after a heavy meal to prevent indigestion – the origin of gingerbread.

How to take it:

Ginger tea (1) Use two teaspoons of the grated root to one cup of boiling water. Let it steep for five minutes. This tea forms a healthy alternative to normal tea or coffee and avoids the intake of caffeine and other stimulants which can act as stressors to the system and so cut down on the ability to perform sexually.

Ginger tea (2) Half a teaspoon of powdered ginger to one cup of boiling water.

Tincture 5–20 drops in any herb tea.

Crystallized ginger Peel and chop a large piece of fresh ginger. Dissolve one cup of sugar in four cups of water. Add the ginger and simmer gently until the root is soft. Leave overnight, drain and pack in sterilized jars.

Cooking Chop into biscuits and cakes, or add to curries.

Ginger ale Make sure it is made with real not synthetic ginger.

Caution: Do not use in cases of high fever, bleeding, inflammatory skin conditions or ulcers. Ginger in large doses can bring on menstruation. Pregnant women with a history of miscarriage should exercise caution and consult their doctor before taking it.

GINKGO BILOBA

Ginkgo biloba, used for centuries in Traditional Chinese Medicine, comes from the maidenhair tree, originally from China and often grown in parks. The tea, tincture and tablets treat a variety of conditions including poor circulation, improving blood flow and strengthening blood vessels – again, potentially good for impotence.

Ginkgo biloba has been the subject of much research by the American Psychiatric Association, among others. Studies indicates that ginkgo biloba improves circulation to the body's extremities such as hands and feet, as well as to the blood vessels that feed the brain – and the same mechanism is also supposed to improve blood flow to the erectile tissues. A preliminary trial of 60 men with erectile dysfunction due to circulation problems reported that half the men regained virility after taking 60mg a day of gingko biloba.

Another study also suggests it may help with sexual difficulties due to taking antidepressants. The men and women, who reported lower libido, were studied for 6–8 weeks on doses from 60–240mg, and found that the gingko biloba supplement did seem to restore desire and performance. They suffered minimal side-effects such as minor stomach problems and lightheadedness.

How to take it:
Tea The tea is said to be best taken in large doses – at least three cups a day for some months.
Tablets Follow the dose on the packet.

GINSENG AND SIBERIAN GINSENG ROOT

Ginseng and Siberan ginseng root (*Panax ginseng* and *Eleutherococcus senticosus*) have been used by oriental men for at least the past 5,000 years as a means of enhancing virility. The word 'ginseng' is said to mean 'the wonder of the world'. In controlled experiments it has been shown to enhance stamina and it probably acts as a general stimulant of the metabolism and general energizer, as well as helping the body cope with stress and strengthening the immune system – all good if loss of sex drive is caused by fatigue or other lifestyle factors. Ginseng may be particularly useful if you use it as a booster while trying to improve your energy in other ways, for example with a better diet.

Ginseng combined with wild yam forms the famous Tigra pill, which sold out within two weeks of it going on sale in France (see separate entry on wild yam, page 55). This is claimed to work on tissue, blood and nerves to enhance sexual arousal.

Ginseng's reputation has rather suffered in recent years, as initially it was often falsely claimed as a miracle herb – and then just as falsely discredited. In fact, ginseng is an adaptogen, which means it supplements any deficiencies in the body, such as sexual energy, and helps the body adapt to different conditions as well as working in conjunction with other herbs and lifestyle factors.

How to take it: 100mg of powdered root or 300mg of cut root in a decoction is the suggested dose, or 20–30 drops of tincture twice daily, but many preparations are available in stores – follow the instructions on the packet.

Tonic wine 1oz/25g powdered ginseng in 2pt/1 litre of red or white wine. Add to taste spices such as cardamon (4 seeds). Stand for two weeks, strain and drink a small glass daily.
Caution: Do not use if pregnant or if you have high blood pressure. May aggravate anxiety and irritability. Do not take large doses in connection with stimulants, or take long-term without professional guidance.

GUARANA

Used by Amazon tribes to keep alert while hunting, guarana is also said to stimulate the sexual appetite. Derived from seeds of the woody liana called *Paullinia cupana*, guarana paste is made from crushed seeds, cassava flour and water, and the paste is then rolled into cylinders and dried. The residue is grated and the shavings dissolved in hot sweet water, with a resulting brew of around 5 per cent caffeine. In about 1870 the explorer Richard Spruce recorded that the Indians of Southern Venezuela drank it first thing in the morning on leaving their hammocks. This drink depends on xanthines for its stimulant effects, which arise because the xanthines increase the production of various secondary messengers within the cells, which leads to a general stimulation of numerous biological processes.
How to take it: Preparations are available from specialist healthcare, healthfood or herbal stores; follow the instructions on the packet.

HORNY GOAT WEED

The aphrodisiac herb horny goat weed, *Epimedium sagittatum*, may sound like a joke, but it has been seriously developed by Dr James Zhou, Associate Scientist at the Faculty Yale School of Medicine and a leading expert on Chinese medicine. Horny goat weed, which grows in the mountains of China, was for many centuries a secret. Horny goat weed is said to be one of the strongest herbs for sexual potency in the entire *Ben Cao* (Ancient Chinese Pharmacopeia). It is supposed to work by increasing sperm count as well as dilating blood capillaries to improve blood flow. In Traditional Chinese Medicine (TCM) terms, it is a 'warm' herb which generates kidney essence, or *jing*, and so nurtures the kidneys, the source, according to Chinese medicine, of many hormonal and reproductive conditions. Jing energy, also called 'essence', is the primordial energy which is given to a person at conception. The closest Western parallel is DNA, our genetic blueprint. Jing energy governs development and growth in the body, and Traditional Chinese Medicine teaches that jing can be strengthened through diet, lifestyle and herbal treatments.

Dr Zhou learned his herbal craft as an apprentice to a Taoist monk, who took him on after his father died as a result of brutal treatment by Mao Zedong's Red Guards. Zhou's own apprenticeship was not without its rough side – part of the training involved banging his hands against a wall and then plunging them into herbal juices so he would not feel the pain. After studying genetics at agricultural school in Beijing, Zhou won a scholarship to Iowa State University and went on to study pharmacology at Yale. His current work is still firmly grounded in his Chinese heritage – his family grow and harvest organic herbs from the mountain plantations in China, and the herbs are processed to Western standards of production in the USA.

Dr Zhou's own formulation uses a mixture of herbs, of which horny goat weed is a very important part. This stems from a belief that a balance of herbs, rather than just one herb, is needed to procure the desired result in cases of sexual difficulty, which so often have a mixture of causes. 'In TCM, sexual impotence has various causes and needs a variety of herbal combinations,' says Dr Zhou. 'A single herb cannot cure impotence. But in precise combination, herbs can enhance sexual energy and performance.' The combinations created by Dr Zhou contain a mix of herbs designed to balance *chi*, the life force according to TCM and also called 'vital energy' or 'primal energy'. TCM practitioners believe that a healthy body is a wellspring of constantly circulating chi which moves round the body and can balance all its functions, including the effects of sexual hormones.

Horny goat weed may be particularly helpful for women with poor sex drive due to fatigue, stress, illness or hormone imbalance, especially in combination with other herbs such as dong quai (see page 57), ginseng (see page 47) and Chinese licorice, a product which works in synergy with the others to help efficacy and absorption. Dr Zhou also uses yohimbe (see page 37) and the combination of herbs helps balance the dilating or widening effects of yohimbe, which works by expanding blood vessels so allowing blood to flow more freely. Dr Zhou believes that a combination of herbs helps people get better results, as they absorb more from a lower dose.

How to take it:

As a tea Preparations are available in specialist health stores. Follow the instructions on the packet.

MUIRA PUAMA

Traditionally used in the Amazon, muira puama, or potency wood, has been used for centuries to soothe the nervous system, increase sexual desire and maintain testosterone levels. It is believed to break down into chemical compounds in the body which tone up tissues in the genital area. Doctors at the Paris Institute of Sexology gave muira puama to 2,000 patients for 10 days and found significant improvement in 60 per cent.

The clinical trials were conducted by Dr Jacques Waynberg, a world authority on sexual function. In the first trial, with 262 patients, 62 per cent of patients with loss of libido claimed the treatment had a perky effect, while 51 per cent with erection failure felt that muira puama was of benefit. The second clinical trial with 100 patients reported that 70 per cent indicated a strengthening of their libido, 66 per cent reported a greater frequency of sex, and 66 per cent reported less fatigue. There were no reported side-effects.

How to take it: Preparations are available in specialist health stores. Follow the instructions on the packet.

NETTLE

The stinging nettle, a common weed found in many countries, has been used for centuries for its medicinal properties – the 16th-century herbalist John Gerard used it as an antidote to poison. It contains iron, which may be very useful in boosting those who are low in energy and so apathetic about sex, especially women as they lose blood through menstruation.

Nettle root is believed to increase free circulating testosterone levels by up to ten times, according to European research reported in 1995. In a clinical study in 1986, it was documented that actual testosterone production does not generally decrease as men age but the amount of free circulating testosterone decreases as more gets bound to the albumin and becomes unavailable for the body's use. Albumin is the most abundant blood protein, synthesized in the liver and present in the blood plasma. Albumin concentrates the blood and attracts water, thereby maintaining the circulatory blood volume. These changes happen during a natural chemical process because of the activity of 'sex hormone binding globulin' or SHBG. Other researchers believe that the increase in SHBG is a major contributing factor in prostate disorders, impotence and a decline in sex drive. Nettles are also rich in chlorophyll and are a source of beta carotene, vitamin C, vitamin E and minerals, especially silica.

How to take it:

Infusion Pick 1oz/25g of young nettle tops and add 1 pint/500ml boiling water. Leave to infuse for 15 minutes for maximum effect.

Decoction Same as preceding entry, but using the root instead of the leaves.

As soup Make a soup with young nettle tops – try adding garlic (see page 43).

RHODIOLA

Rhodiola rosea, the Arctic root, is said to be a versatile herb with many benefits, and was found by a Russian botanist in 1931 to enhance sexual potency and physical endurance. It also increases resistance to stress. Soviet scientists continued to research this native plant and decided that, like the more famous ginseng, it is an adaptogen or compound that helps build what the individual body needs. Research suggests rhodiola may protect chemical messengers (neurotransmitters) in the brain from toxins such as serotonin which calm and elevate mood. Rhodiola is believed to improve neurotransmitter activity by combating potentially harmful enzymes and preventing the release of too much stress hormones by the adrenal glands. It can also increase serotonin by up to 30 per cent, according to studies.

How to take it: Preparations are available in specialist health or herbal stores. Follow the instructions on the packet.

SARSAPARILLA

Sarsaparilla has a worldwide reputation and history of use, dating back to the 1600s, as an aphrodisiac and male tonic. Said to to increase testosterone levels, it was particularly well known to the Indians of Mexico and South America who used it as a tonic for general weakness as well as to improve sexual performance. They also used it for rheumatism and skin problems. John Gerard recommends it for 'continual aches and pains in the joints and against cold diseases'.

Sarsaparilla has been found to contain the hormones testosterone, progesterone and cortin, which helps explain sarsaparilla's use as a sexual stimulant. Dr Emerick Solomo, a Hungarian scientist living in Mexico, did several tests with sarsaparilla root on thousands of animals and men, and concluded that the hormones in sarsaparilla do benefit their users by strengthening those who take it and so improving their sexual function.

How to take it: Preparations are available in specialist health or herbal stores. Follow the instructions on the packet.

SAW PALMETTO (SERENOA SERRULATA)

Saw palmetto, a small, palm-like plant, can be found in sand dunes along the Atlantic and Caribbean coasts. Its berries have long held a reputation as a sexual stimulant – it is supposed to work directly on the sex hormones. It is also known as the 'plant catheter' due to its therapeutic effect on the bladder and the prostate in men, and it helps maintain prostate health by balancing oestrogen levels which could otherwise interact negatively with the gland's tissues. Saw palmetto extract works to prevent testosterone from converting into dihydrotestosterone, the hormone thought to cause prostate cells to multiply, leading to an enlarged prostate. Saw palmetto inhibits androgen and oestrogen receptor activity and may be beneficial for both sexes in balancing the hormones. Because of its hormonal effects, saw palmetto is also believed to help the thyroid in regulating sexual development.

Native Americans and early American settlers used the berries to treat problems in the genitals, urinary tract and reproductive system. Today, it is still widely used in Germany, Canada, the United Kingdom and the US to treat problems of the prostate and urinary tract, with the main uses being as a supplement for reducing enlarged prostate glands, treating urinary tract problems and for improving general strength. It has also been used for thyroid deficiency, chest congestion, coughs, asthma and bronchitis, as well as to stimulate appetite, improve digestion, nourish the nervous system and increase the assimilation of nutrients by the body.

In addition, it is renowned as an aphrodisiac and tonic. Saw palmetto is one of the few herbal remedies that are considered to be anabolic, strengthening and building body tissues. The active constituents are volatile oil, steroidal saponin, tannins and polysaccharides. Steroidal saponins are structurally similar to human sex and stress hormones. These hormone-like saponins resemble cholesterol, cortisone, oestrogen, progesterone and vitamin D.

Women have used the herb to stimulate breast enlargement and lactation as well as treating ovarian and uterine irritability. It has been prescribed for reduced or absent sex drive, impotence and frigidity.

How to take it:

Decoction Half a teaspoon of the crushed berries to one cup of water. Drink one or two cups a day.

Tincture Available from specialist herb stores. Take 20–40 drops, in water, three times a day.

With nettle root Chop two or three handfuls of fresh nettle root. Place in a jar and cover with saw palmetto tincture. Leave for two weeks, shaking from time to time. Strain and bottle. Take 30 drops three times a day. This is especially effective for prostate problems.
Caution: Because of its potential hormonal effects, saw palmetto should not be used during pregnancy. Always have suspected prostate problems medically checked.

WILD YAM

Wild yam, or *Dioscorea villosa*, is the rhizome of the Mexican wild yam, and it has been known for its aphrodisiac qualities to witch-doctors or *cuaranderos* in Mexico for many centuries. The dried root, which retains its medicinal properties for over a year, is also said to be anti-inflammatory and anti-spasmodic, and is the starting point for synthesization of hormones for the contraceptive pill and for natural progesterone used in a cream for women at the menopause.
How to take it: Preparations are available in specialist health or herbal stores. Follow the instructions on the packet.
Decoction Half a teaspoon of the grated root to one cup water. Drink one or two cups a day.

Visiting a herbalist

A herbalist will look at your overall health and wellbeing and will be able to create a mixture of ingredients individually tailored to your particular needs, and which takes account of any other weaknesses or imbalances in your system. Many herbalists believe that, while the use of 'simples' (single herbs) has a place, it is often the combination

AYURVEDIC MEDICINE

AYURVEDA IS AN ANCIENT HEALING tradition from India that dates back at least 5,000 years, and is the art of living in harmony with Nature and her laws in order to promote maximum health and wellbeing. Like other natural systems of medicine, Ayurvedic medicine focuses on holistic aspects of treatment. According to Ayurveda, problems such as low libido have to be considered in the overall context of a person's life – disorders and illnesses represent the end of a long, ongoing process which is the natural expression of a person's life, and it is no good treating just the symptoms and ignoring the person. From this viewpoint, low libido may be a psychologically healthy protest at an unsatisfactory relationship. Or, according to Dr Vasant Lad, a world-renowned expert on Ayurvedic studies (see Further Reading), it may be a sign of the 'body's intelligence' in that the body shuts down sexually so as to conserve energy in times of low vitality or health – or to expend that energy on other creative areas. So, when trying herbal remedies, try and ensure that other areas of your life are in balance, too. According to Dr Lad, low libido and impotence can be helped by several herbal remedies. You can consult a practitioner, which may be wise if you suffer from severe sexual dysfunction, but many of these remedies can easily be used at home, especially if it's just a case of raising libido that little bit extra.

HERBAL REMEDIES For impotence, Dr Lad recommends taking a mixture of equal parts (a quarter to a half a teaspoon each) of ***ashwagandha***, ***bala*** and ***vidari***, all viewed as strengthening herbs in Ayurvedic medicine. One teaspoon of this mixture is taken twice a day in warm milk for three months. A few pieces of chopped fresh garlic can be added, which improves the blood supply and helps the blood vessels dilate so that blood flow is improved.

FOR WOMEN Use the boosting herb ***shatavari*** instead of ***ashwagandha***. Mix one teaspoon ***shatavari*** with half a teaspoon ***vidari*** and take it with a cup of warm milk at night before going to bed.

TRANQUILLITY TEA If you think the root of your impotence is psychological, for example due to anxiety or stress, you may be able to correct this by drinking a tea made up of the soothing herbs, ***jatamamsi*, *brahmi*** and ***shanka pushpi*** in equal proportions (a quarter to a half a teaspoon each). Make a tea from half a teaspoon of this mixture, and drink it about an hour before going to bed. It is said definitely to help with any emotional or psychological stress which may be at the root of sexual problems and so may be good for both men and women.

SPICED DRINKS Another Ayurvedic option is a mild aphrodisiac drink of warm milk with a pinch of saffron – saffron is an aphrodisiac for men and women, and increases sperm count.

These herbs are available from a good natural food store, some Indian groceries, or via specialist Ayurveda health centres (see Useful Addresses).

of herbs which is key to successful treatment, and that herbs will work in different ways depending on what they are mixed with. The herbalist will also be able to prescribe the right dosage for you – many people try herbs for themselves and give up in dissatisfaction simply because they have taken too little or too much of the herb. It is important to inform the herbalist if you are pregnant or know you have a health condition.

Herbalists vary in what they may prescribe, and prescriptions will vary from person to person, but might include the following:

- Lobelia – a relaxant.
- Cayenne – to regulate high blood pressure and increase blood flow.
- St John's Wort, or *Hypericum perforatum* – stress depletes the libido and this well-known anti-stress herb encourages physical

Traditional Chinese Medicine

IN TRADITIONAL CHINESE MEDICINE (TCM), Chinese doctors treat the body as a whole rather than just treating impotence, which they believe is a sign that kidney energy is low. TCM describes sexual dysfunction as originating in the brain, and then flowing to the reproductive organs via the kidneys – healthy kidneys are linked with the healthy functioning of the adrenal and reproductive organs. A Chinese doctor will use a range of herbs which might include for example cnidium, believed to warm the kidneys and traditionally used for impotence, and cinnamon bark, which helps regulate stimulation. Another herb often used by Western herbalists as well as Chinese practitioners is dong quai. Sometimes known as Chinese angelica or the 'female ginseng', this herb is traditionally regarded as being especially for women. Dong quai is believed to have a balancing effect on women's hormonal systems, and to act as an all-purpose sexual and reproductive tonic.

and mental relaxation and feelings of wellbeing, as well as countering depression.

- Other herbs recommended singly or, more often in combination include *Serenoa repens*, pumpkin seed, passion flower, hawthorn, *Turnera aphrodisiaca* leaf, wild yam root, ma huang, orchid, and *Aletris farinosa* (true unicorn root).

CHAPTER THREE

How to Help Yourself: Lifestyle Changes

SEX may often seem to have a life of its own, but as already pointed out, it is definitely linked to the rest of the body's wellbeing. Much of the joy of sex is linked to optimal health, which is within most people's reach with a little effort. Simple lifestyle changes can often be powerful and effective ways to restore sexuality, and you may be amazed at how easily and quickly low libido vanishes once you start making improvements in areas such as diet, exercise and relaxation. All of these measures may also be able to help more severe sexual dysfunction too, and they're not gender-restricted – they work for both men and women.

The results can be profound, and may extend far beyond sexual performance. The links between lifestyle and health are being increasingly recognized both by the medical profession and people in general, and healthy living, as a tool which can prevent as well as heal disease, is set to carry us into the 21st century. Paying attention to lifestyle can help keep you young, boost and cleanse your whole system and give your skin and other organs a general work-out which will leave you feeling totally refreshed, relaxed and energetic. You may find that many common ailments magically vanish – the headaches, the pre-menstrual tension, the tiredness and all the little and bigger niggles which we so often take for granted as part of life. The classic excuse

'Not tonight – I've got a headache' may become a thing of the past!

The right lifestyle can leave you mentally more alert, encouraging motivation and balance and restoring awareness and creativity. You may find yourself better equipped to deal with modern-day stress, anxiety and tension. Emotionally, too, depression and mood swings are likely to ease up significantly as you learn to listen to your body and give it what it needs in terms of rest, cleansing, activity and nourishment.

You don't have to be a health fanatic to achieve all this – many of the suggested lifestyle changes in this chapter are within easy reach of everyone. But, even if some of them do take a little effort, it will be worth it. The more relaxed, healthy and confident you are, the more alluring you are, and the more easy and natural you will find it to enjoy what your body, and that of your partner, has to offer.

Is your diet adequate?

Lowered sex drive and sexual dysfunction can both be symptoms of a diet which is lacking in certain vitamins and minerals, as much research has shown. Loss of sexual desire, as well as many of the of the symptoms listed below, was noted by researchers at the University of Minnesota who looked at people with insufficient diets, including those lacking protein and B vitamins.

Have a look at the items in the following list, all of which can be signs that your diet is inadequate. (They may also be symptoms of some other underlying disorder, so if in doubt, consult your doctor.)

- tiredness and weakness
- irritability

- feeling more introverted and lacking interest in others
- lack of interest in personal appearance
- anxiety
- melancholy
- morbidity
- depression symptoms such as problems sleeping, especially early morning waking, and weight changes
- slowing down mentally and physically
- loss of interest in your surroundings, house, clothes, appearance
- bursting into tears
- feeling unworthy
- feeling unable to cope
- feeling life isn't worth living
- difficulty in concentrating
- decreased ability to work
- cold hands and feet.

Healthy eating

Although certain foods have been linked with sexual performance for centuries, there has been a revolution in the way we consider diet and health over the past decade or so. It is increasingly being acknowledged that how we eat affects how we live, sleep and die, as well as how we make love. Diet has many proven links with allergy, and with illnesses such as cancer, heart disease and diabetes. Small wonder then that the right diet can make an enormous difference to the health of the sexual organs, and men in particular are well advised to consider their prostate when choosing food and drink because of the rise in prostate cancer (see page 68). As well as keeping the sex organs in the peak of health, the right diet can boost flagging desire.

Specialist advice can also make radical differences to health – for example if you're debilitated due to poor diet, or suffer severe allergies or intolerances to certain foods. More generally, however, we would all benefit from following some simple guidelines.

- ***Don't miss breakfast.*** Having breakfast may actually set the scene for passion later on at night, because breakfast wakes your metabolism up and will help prevent dips in blood sugar which could otherwise lead to that 'I'm too tired tonight' feeling. It is also healthier in terms of processing calories and maintaining weight – research shows that you are more likely to burn off up to 200 calories consumed at breakfast than the same amount consumed later in the day – so is more likely to make you feel slim and sexy!
- ***Keep that blood sugar boosted.*** Plan main meals around unrefined complex carbohydrates such as wholemeal pasta, brown rice and potatoes, so that your energy is maintained right up to bedtime. Look at the section on sexy nutrients below for ideas on sauces to accompany them. For example, seafood sauce is rich in zinc and other important minerals, while vegetable curry contains many nutrients important to sexual health. Cut down on all sources of sugar such as sweets, biscuits and cakes – these only cause quick surges in energy, followed by equally quick drops.
- ***Boost your blood flow.*** Bearing in mind the importance of good circulation, especially for male performance, cut back on red meats which contain a lot of artery-clogging saturated fats, and eat chicken, white fish or oily fish instead. To cook these, grill, bake, or fry with two tablespoons of water, rather than fry in oil. Also cut down on salt.
- ***Eat a variety of foods.*** This common dietary advice has particular

relevance when it comes to sex, because the more varied your diet, the more likely you are to have enough of all the nutrients whose lack can sometimes cause low libido, such as the B vitamins and magnesium (see Sexy Nutrients below).

- ***Think colour.*** Go for lots of colour when choosing vegetables. Yellow, red and green vegetables such as peppers, broccoli and spinach all contain antioxidants which absorb free radicals and so reduce the risk of heart disease, a particularly common source of impotence in men.
- ***Keep the calories up.*** While slim may be sexy, if you're trying too hard to diet, lack of calories can sometimes make you lethargic and/or irritable, and research has shown that calorie restriction is one of the first things which will destroy sex drive. Rather than trying to restrict calories so you're uncomfortable, it's better to try and aim for healthy eating habits so you feel more energetic.

What to eat – sexy nutrients

According to Dr Sarah Brewer, a British general and sexual health expert, certain nutrients are specifically linked with sexual and reproductive health, as well as being generally good for you. Nutrients may help maintain a healthy balance of sex and other hormones, or boost your health and energy generally with subsequent beneficial effects on your sex life.

- ***Protein.*** Studies have shown that lack of protein causes libido to fall and sperm count to lessen, as well as causing apathy and lack of energy. Sources of protein include soya (including tofu), quinoa, beans, lentils, meat, eggs, fish and dairy products.

- ***Essential fatty acids.*** These are needed to help form the male sex hormone testosterone. Good sources include seeds (flax seed or linseed, sunflower, sesame, pumpkin), and cold-pressed seed oils.
- ***B vitamins.*** Vitamin B6 regulates sex-hormone function and men lacking vitamin B6 have become impotent. Vitamin B3 (niacin) helps improve circulation and is necessary for the production of certain hormones, so much so that it has been described as an aphrodisiac. Lack of B vitamins in general can create fatigue, depression, irritability, apathy and anxiety, among many other un-sexy symptoms. Good sources include yeast, liver, wheatgerm, meat, yeast extract, fortified cereals, bread and Brussels sprouts.
- ***Vitamin C.*** This is vital for overall and sexual health, and helps strengthen the sexual organs in men and women. Offering protection against cancer and heart disease, vitamin C strengthens the immune system and also helps fight stress. Sources include citrus fruit, blackcurrants, peppers, potatoes, watercress, cabbage, cauliflower, strawberries and tomatoes.
- ***Vitamin D.*** This is vital for bone health as it helps the body retain and process calcium. Deficiency can cause joint pain, backache and muscle cramps, none of which make for spontaneous sex. Vitamin D is made in the skin, which is why exposure to sunlight is our major source. However, food sources include oily fish such as herrings, mackerel and salmon, as well as oysters, cottage cheese and eggs.
- ***Iron.*** Iron boosts your haemoglobin levels, as well as general and sexual energy, and deficiency can cause apathy, fatigue and listlessness. Good sources include red meat, bread, flour, egg yolk, dried fruit, watercress, pumpkin seeds, parsley, almonds, prunes and raisins.
- ***Magnesium.*** Magnesium is one of those key minerals which performs many functions, including regulating the function of heart and other muscles and the nervous system by helping provide the necessary

overall bodily co-ordination for sexual function. People lacking magnesium suffer nervousness and irritability. Good sources include wheatgerm, soya beans, nuts, buckwheat flour and other wholegrains, seafood, dairy products, bananas and dark-green leafy vegetables.

- ***Calcium.*** A lack of calcium creates nervous tension and irritability, neither of which are conducive to closeness. Good sources of calcium include dairy products, bony fish like sardines, bread, green vegetables, baked beans and figs.
- ***Manganese.*** This is essential for healthy sexual function and sources include black tea, wholegrains, watercress, pineapple, blackberries and other fruit, nuts, seeds, eggs, seafood and vegetables.
- ***Selenium.*** Selenium helps regulate the sex hormones by boosting the action of vitamin E which is needed to maintain the male reproductive system. Deficiency signs include high blood pressure and frequent infections. Sources include broccoli, mushrooms, molasses, cabbage, garlic, wholegrains, nuts, seafood such as tuna, oysters and herrings.
- ***Boron.*** This mineral helps the body use calcium and may stimulate energy and sexual appetite. Sources include strawberries, peaches and mangoes.
- ***Phosphorus.*** New research suggests that this mineral can increase sex drive and responsiveness. Good sources of phosphorus include seafood (especially crabmeat and lobster), truffles, eggs, wheatgerm, wheat bran, legumes and seeds (which may explain the traditional Eastern European affection for seeds and nuts as aphrodisiacs).

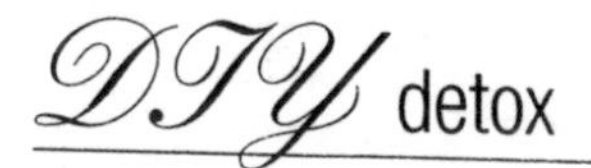

detox

Toxins are everywhere – in air, water and food – but the right diet can to some extent protect against them. Detoxification aims to rid the body of

SUPER-SEXY NUTRIENTS

ZINC

OYSTERS ARE RENOWNED as an aphrodisiac, especially with a glass or so of champagne to help them slip down. Oysters are rich in zinc, an antioxidant mineral which is important to sexual health as it helps regulate the sex hormone testosterone and semen levels.

Semen contains relatively large amounts of zinc, 5mg of which is lost with each ejaculation (around one third of the recommended daily intake). It is believed that zinc helps protect the genetic make-up of sperm and makes for stronger, more energetic sperm. Lack of zinc before adolescence can delay sexual development and can result in smaller male sex organs, and low libido and sexual dysfunction. This obviously applies to men but some experts believe that women with zinc deficiency may also suffer loss of desire too as zinc plays such an important part in balancing the sex hormones, and also helps to maintain vaginal lubrication.

Due to modern food processing, the average diet may be deficient in zinc, and stress, caffeine, smoking and alcohol all increase the need for zinc. Good sources of zinc, apart from oysters, include other seafood, red meat, wholegrains, pulses, eggs, cheese, peanuts, sunflower seeds, oatmeal, yeast and milk.

VITAMIN E

VITAMIN E HAS BEEN SPECIFICALLY RECOMMENDED as a supplement to combat impotence, and has been tested as a treatment for subfertility, and may well be among the ingredients in supplements you see labelled 'for men'. Like zinc, vitamin E is implicated in sexual health, and the quality of sperm bears a direct relation to the amount of vitamin E in a man's semen. Without vitamin E, the testicles of animals have been shown to degenerate and there is a decrease in sex hormones.

In both men and women, vitamin F also protects the sex hormones from destruction by oxygen, strengthens muscle fibres and helps absorb potentially harmful free radicals. It's best taken accompanied by vitamin C to help activate it. Good sources include vegetables, margarine, eggs, butter and wheatgerm.

toxins and impurities which slow it down and make it sluggish and unresponsive to sex. A detox offers a wonderful opportunity to let your body swing into its own self-healing mode, as you take a day or two in which you relax, consume simple, cleansing food and drink, and allow your body to renew and recharge itself. A detox rests the digestive system, significant when you think that the digestive process normally uses up to 30 per cent of our energy. By allowing it time off, you help re-direct the body's energy to where it is most needed – in this case, the sexual organs. Detoxing has also been recommended as a cure for listlessness and stress. At its most rigorous, and perhaps successful, it is probably best done under expert guidance, so you may want to consult a nutritionist who specializes in this area. An expert may perform specific tests such as iridology or vega which will pinpoint particular imbalances, and then certain nutrients will be suggested according to the results. However, it is easy to do a general detox yourself, and health expert and author Marie Farquharson suggests a programme which will leave you relaxed, revitalized, and more tuned in to your body's physical and emotional needs.

TWO DAY JUICE FAST (FRUIT AND VEGETABLE)

Fruit juices cleanse the blood while vegetable juices build and regenerate it. This combination uses the best of both worlds, with nutrient-rich liquids which are digested within minutes of being drunk, so giving your digestive system a holiday.

Two weeks before

- Book two days off.
- Detox your home to remove any 'stuck' energy – throw out or

The prostate

THE PROSTATE GLAND is vital to reproductive and general health in men. Usually described as being the size of a chestnut, it is situated below the base of the bladder, surrounding the urethra. The prostate secretes fluids that make up to 40 per cent of semen volume, directs semen outward during ejaculation and makes prostaglandins (hormone-like substances). If the prostate becomes enlarged or inflamed, it can cause painful urination and ejaculation. It is estimated that men between 20 and 50 have a one-in-three chance of developing prostatis, or inflammation of the prostate, while the incidence of prostate cancer is soaring and looks set to overtake that of lung and breast cancer in the UK, according to the Institute of Cancer Research. So, it does make sense to take care of the prostate – you will be looking after your long-term health as well as your sexuality by doing so.

TIPS FOR A HEALTHY PROSTATE

- *Eat a low-fat diet*, especially Eastern style. Japanese men, who traditionally eat a low-fat, soya-rich diet, have a lower incidence of prostate cancer. So, go for a diet which includes rice and cruciferous vegetables (cabbage, turnip, kohlrabi, Chinese leaves) which contain plant hormones such as isoflavonoids and phytoestrogens which can protect against some diseases and cancers. Also eat soya products such as beans, tofu and soya sauce. Soya helps to balance hormone levels, disruption of which is believed to cause some cancers.
- *Eat organic meat and dairy products* where possible to avoid foods with a high hormone content.
- *Choose foods to help prostate function*. Foods said to be good for the prostate include pumpkin and sesame seeds, a rich source of essential fatty acids. Also eat foods rich in vitamin E, selenium and zinc (see pages 65 and 66).
- *Saw palmetto* (see page 53), is often recommended for prostate disorders.
- *Avoid violent exercise* when the bladder is full as any urine which spills over into the gland can cause inflammation.
- *Practise yoga exercises*. Certain yoga positions may help strengthen the prostate and improve sexual function.

organize clutter and have a spring clean. This stems from feng shui principles, according to which every space has an energy which affects you physically and emotionally.

- Start running down your supplies of non-detox-friendly food (such as processed meats and fish, convenience foods, cans, packet and ready-made meals and sugary products such as cakes and biscuits).

One week before

- Start to cut down or exclude refined foods, animal products (meat, fish, eggs and dairy produce) as well as alcohol, tea, coffee and cigarettes, while boosting your intake of fruits, vegetables, nuts, grains and seeds. Drink water and herb teas. This will get your body into peak working condition and help cut down on toxins in the first place.
- Book yourself in for a massage, sauna or steam bath for the afternoon of your first day.
- Start shopping for the fresh fruit and vegetables you will need (organic if possible) towards the end of the week.

The day before

- If you haven't done so already, cut out the foods mentioned in the last section. If you smoke, try and stop completely. Also cut out alcohol.
- In the evening, eat a light meal such as a green salad with olive-oil dressing or a vegetable soup.
- Plan how to deal with outside interruptions over the next couple of days. The fewer interruptions you have the better, so leave the answering machine on or unplug the phone.

- Start to focus your thoughts on the next day or two, have a warm bath and go to bed early.

Day one/two

(The programme is the same for both days.)

- ***Generally:*** have a slow, relaxed start to the day, and keep it that way, including yoga, meditation, breathing exercises, walks, baths or whatever you fancy to help you tune in to your body and yourself – this is *your* two days, when you devote time to yourself. Be sure to drink plenty of fluids – as well as the liquid recommended below, top up with still mineral or spring water, aiming to drink about three and a half to six pints (two to three and a half litres) to help flush the toxins out of your body.
- ***On waking:*** drink a glass of warm water with the juice of half a lemon.
- ***Breakfast:*** one apple, two pears, half a pineapple, peeled, juiced and mixed. Mix with mineral water if you find it too strong.
- ***Lunch:*** one apple, two carrots, half a galia melon, 1cm fresh ginger root, juiced and mixed.
- ***Afternoon:*** go for a massage – or get your partner to give you one at home.
- ***Evening meal:*** four carrots, four tomatoes, small bunch of parsley, juiced.
- ***Around 9p.m.:*** drink a glass of warm water with lemon juice or ginger, and go to bed.

(Adapted from *Natural Detox* by Marie Farquharson, Element Books, 1999.)

Exercise

Like diet, exercise can be the factor that tips people into good sexual health. Its benefits are many and general – it improves strength and stamina, reduces cholesterol and reduces the risk of osteoporosis (thinning bones) in later life.

More particularly, exercise helps combat many of the mild or more serious disorders which can impair performance. Exercise is dramatically good for your heart and circulation, which as we have seen are closely implicated in good sexual performance. Regular, vigorous exercise can cut the risk of heart disease by half, and also reduces high blood pressure. It may well banish low libido and make substantial advances towards helping more severe sexual dysfunction, but do give it time to work (2–3 weeks), and for your body to absorb its beneficial effects.

Exercise also helps combat stress, which lowers levels of sex hormones and sexual desire. Exercise releases endorphins, the body's natural 'feel-good' substances, stretches tense muscles and leaves them – and you – more relaxed. Exercise can also be key in boosting physical confidence, something which can easily dwindle if you feel your sexual performance is less than adequate.

Obesity, also linked with low sex drive and poor performance, can be helped by exercise, especially when combined with good nutrition. Exercise alone may only result in a smallish calorie loss – around 300 calories (two pieces of toast) for running a mile. But done every day, that's 9,300 calories a month – a weight loss approaching 5lb (2¼kg). Exercise also speeds up your metabolic rate, helping you process food more efficiently, and it has also been shown that moderate exercise actually makes you less hungry as it activates appetite-regulating mechanisms in the body.

The incidence of another key underlying condition which makes impotence more likely, diabetes, can also be reduced with exercise. One study of nearly 6,000 men found that regular exercise cut the risk of diabetes irrespective of how overweight the men were. Another massive study of nearly 90,000 women showed that vigorous exercise at least once a week reduced the risk of diabetes by a third. It is believed that exercise works against diabetes by increasing insulin sensitivity and so helping keep blood sugar levels steady.

Small, regular amounts of exercise seem to be better than great long exhausting bursts as they are more effective in getting your heart to work properly. The usual recommended amount is 15–20 minutes three times a week. But, whatever you can manage is good. It's also effective to build more physical activity into your daily activities, so that you walk to work or the shops instead of taking the car, use the stairs instead of the lift and so on. Even small amounts will help you build an 'exercise mentality' so that you gradually come to depend more on the good effects of exercise – the re-energizing glow after brisk walking, or the general feeling of relaxation after a swim.

Alcohol

From Bacchanalian rites to modern-day happy hours, alcohol has been used as an aphrodisiac. In 405 BC, the Greek playwright Euripides observed, 'And if wine ceases, there will be an end of Love, an end to every pleasure in the life of man.' Centuries later, Shakespeare more cynically observed that although alcohol 'provokes the desire' it also 'takes away the performance'.

There is a widespread belief in the power of alcohol to enhance pleasure. A survey of 20,000 people by the journal *Psychology Today* found that around two in three women and nearly one in two men believe that alcohol enhances sexual pleasure. But is it truly an aphrodisiac?

A glass or two can certainly raise confidence and make you feel sexier and less inhibited. But medical research shows clearly that after the first four to five units (see page 74), alcohol works against erectile powers in men. It stops being a stimulant and starts being a depressant, acting on the heart and respiratory system and so lowering the ability to perform, sometimes resulting in the dreaded 'brewer's droop'. In fact, drinking alcohol is thought to cause one in six cases of erectile dysfunction.

Acetaldehyde, produced when alcohol breaks down in the body, is actually a poison for living cells and can cause damage to the liver, brain and heart. Overindulgence in alcohol can result in fatty liver degeneration, which in turn causes a drop in testosterone levels and so drops in sex drive and sperm counts – the enzymes that break down alcohol also break down the male hormone.

Red wine has acquired a reputation for being good for your heart, and several international studies have found that a moderate intake can reduce the risk of heart attack by as much as 40 per cent. However, you don't have to drink alcohol to get the good effects – red grape juice and alcohol-free red wine also contain antioxidants which are thought to help keep arteries clear and prevent them clogging up. It should also be noted that too much red wine, like other forms of alcohol, can cause high blood pressure, lowered testosterone levels, lower sex drive and low sperm count.

But, in moderate amounts, alcohol seems to work very effectively on one organ – the brain. Whether the effect is due to changes in body chemistry or changes in perception, limited drinking may be a useful ice-breaker in sexual situations. Research does hint that faith in the sexual power of alcohol makes you believe you are more sexually aroused, regardless of the physical facts. In at least three studies, women reported increasing sexual pleasure as their blood alcohol level increased, despite a decreased volume of blood that should have lessened sexual feeling. Even as sexual activity declined with drinking, 69 women who kept diaries of their sexual experiences reported that drinking enhanced their desire. So, while the aphrodisiac effect of alcohol can't really be proven, perhaps the subjective approach is best. If you believe alcohol makes you feel sexier, you will probably live up to it!

Smoking

Cigarettes are one of the biggest causes of erectile dysfunction and other sexual problems – just two cigarettes smoked before sex will markedly decrease the blood flow to the penis. And, there is definitely a dose-related effect – that is, the more you smoke, the less likely you are to have sex.

Alcohol units

1 UNIT ALCOHOL =

- 100ml/one glass of wine
- 50ml/one measure of sherry
- 25ml/one measure spirit
- 300ml/half pint beer or cider

The slowing of blood flow may also affect women, with decreased blood flow to the genital area.

Because of the damaging effect on circulation smoking ultimately causes cardiovascular diseases such as arteriosclerosis (clogging of the arteries) which affects blood flow – vital for effective erection. You may not even stay alive to enjoy half the sex which your lifespan seemed to promise – a study of half a million smokers proved that the risk of premature death is nearly twice as high in smokers than in non-smokers. All this is quite apart from the immediate cosmetic effects such as skin and hair odour.

It takes from four to eight weeks to start feeling the health benefits of stopping smoking, as your circulation improves. According to Dr Sarah Brewer, after this time the male sperm count increases significantly and erections become more rigid.

GIVING UP

Giving up nicotine is notoriously difficult – some say even harder than giving up drink and drugs – but it can be done. The key to success is getting support. Doing it alone is possible, but good, consistent support will make the process easier and more likely to be successful in the long run. Support can help maintain motivation in the face of temptation, pick you up after a fall and help you slowly create a lifestyle in which smoking just doesn't play a part.

- First look at your immediate circle of friends and family. Is it a 'smoking culture'? If so, you may need more support to help break the habit, so consider contacting a support organization such as ASH in the UK who can offer well-researched and practical advice.
- Make the decision, either now or at a certain set time when you feel it

would be easier, so you can work yourself into the right state of mind.

- Write 10 affirmations two or three times a day around giving up, such as 'I, (name), can give up smoking.' If you like, add a limited time: '(name) won't have a cigarette this morning/for the next hour/five minutes.' This helps break the day down into more manageable units.
- Generally, take short-term views. Just try and get through the morning.
- Break old smoking associations – get rid of smoking accessories such as ashtrays, lighters and so on, and avoid situations where you've always smoked, such as the pub. This can be hard if you realize that smoking is inextricably bound up with your social life, and that abandoning one means a void in the other. However, it doesn't have to be for ever, and meanwhile seek out your helpful, rather than unhelpful friends, maybe exploring other social avenues such as, perhaps, a meditation class.
- Hypnotherapy may be worth a try as it is one of the most effective cures for smoking.

Stress and relaxation

Stress is a notorious libido-killer as it releases adrenalin, a hormone which in small doses might help you catch a mate, but too much of which sends the body into red alert and unable to relax sufficiently for lovemaking. Adrenalin raises blood sugar levels to provide energy for the well-known 'fight or flight' response. The circulation to some parts of the body shuts down so more blood can go to the muscles, and the testicles are drawn safely up to the abdomen.

As well as lowered sex drive and impotence, the physical effects of stress include:

- sweating
- flushing
- palpitations
- dizziness
- pins and needles
- stomach pain
- ulcers
- nausea
- insomnia
- high blood pressure
- depressed immunity with lowered resistance to infections, stroke, angina, heart attack and even cancer.

And the mental effects include:

- anxiety
- panic
- inability to cope
- fear of failure and rejection
- inability to concentrate
- drinking too much
- smoking or taking drugs, obsessive or compulsive behaviour, feeling isolated or having a feeling of impending doom.

Recreational drugs

VARIOUS RECREATIONAL DRUGS such as alcohol might seem to promise sexual enhancement but tend not to live up to their promise.

- One of the effects of cannabis is slight engorgment of the genitals, as well as the well-known euphoria and heightened perception of colour, objects and time. It also helps people relax so is an attractive option for first-night nerves – but it can also relax the parts that drugs should not reach. It also slows reflexes and other motor activity. Take too much, and you may have a pleasant, laid-back night with absolutely no physical contact at all.
- Cocaine and crack also promise great 'highs', including increased sexual excitement, but their ability to decrease erection reflects the milder end of a stream of unsexy health effects which range from a running and bleeding nose to irregularity of the heartbeat and epileptic-type seizures.

DEALING WITH STRESS

Most stress comes from within. Although some situations are inherently more stressful than others, it is our reaction which is key. It is also often possible to take action to lessen outside stresses.

- Set clear, but manageable goals – confusion about aims can cause stress.
- Write affirmations to help create a positive self-image as constant worrying about your self-worth is stressful.
- Work out what situations and people cause you stress and why.
- Now write down where you can change matters and take some action no matter how small.

WHAT ABOUT ANGER?

ANGER is a very natural response both to stress and to sexual difficulties, but anger can also be a major inhibitor of sexual response.

Interestingly, there is little difference between the physiological states of anger and of sexual arousal, as well-known UK therapist Gael Lindelfield points out: according to research, there are fourteen similar changes and only four differences in the two states! So, holding back anger may also mean holding back on sexual expression, and managing anger may be key in releasing, accepting and managing sexual satisfaction. Men may feel angry because social stereotypes dictate that they should always be virile and ready for sex, while women may try and repress anger at being deprived of sex because tradition equally dictates that they are not really supposed to feel lust, and should place caring for others before personal satisfaction.

Managing stress may be key in managing the anger which can cut off sexual responses, along with other benefits, such as greater self-assertiveness, improved communication and more positive thinking.

- Accept there are certain situtions where you may not be in control, i.e. changes in relationships, work. Allow yourself to make mistakes.
- Allow yourself time to make decisions. Remember there are three ways to do this – either/or, the middle route, or 'taken under further consideration'. Give your unconscious mind a chance to come up with a solution. If necessary, 'sleep on it'.
- Work sensible hours and ensure you take time off to relax.
- Sleep enough (see page 83).
- Get fit.
- Avoid coffeee, tea and alcohol.
- Meditate to overcome what Deepak Chopra calls 'the disease of being in a hurry'. In conversation, breathe deeply and pause before replying, to give yourself time to think and to avoid interrupting.

BACK PAIN

BACK PAIN, comic token of a fulfilled sexual relationship, can actually cause serious sexual problems between couples. They may see each other using the pain as an excuse not to have sex, so that the way back pain impacts on relationships can be major, yet is all too often ignored. Sufferers may find sex intensely awkward or painful, but feel guilty about avoiding it, while partners may equally feel guilty for wanting sex and causing pain, and angry at being denied. Conventional medicine may often have limitations when it comes to addressing back pain. Physiotherapist Lauren Hebert, who has been treating back pain sufferers for more than 20 years in Maine, USA, wrote a book called ***Sex and Back Pain*** (see Further Reading) on realizing what a common problem this is. This uses exercises based on roughly the two main categories into which back problems fall. Flexion principle means it hurts less to bend forward (flexion) than backward. Extension principle means it hurts less to bend backwards (extension) than forward.

Other altemative remedies you can try for back pain include the Alexander Technique and Yoga – see Chapter 4.

Let's talk about it

Unspoken feelings can be key in blocking sexual expression, especially in men who traditionally have more problems in expressing their feelings, seeking solace in the pub or via sports rather than in discussion with friends. However, male emotional health is a vital component of overall sexual health. 'Men are twice as likely to commit suicide than women, which suggests that they tend to neglect their emotional as well as their physical health,' says Dr Steve Carroll, international healthcare consultant and author. Men also are very prone to give up trying at sex if they suffer erectile failure a few times in a row, and then to suffer in silence.

Men's general health awareness remains a major challenge. Men have a much higher risk of dying young from a preventable condition, such as heart disease, stroke and some cancers. In a survey by the UK magazine *Men's Health*, as part of their ongoing UK National Men's Health Awareness Campaign, the 5,000 men surveyed tended to be much more reluctant than women to visit a doctor, even to have persistent symptoms diagnosed. Ninety-one per cent said they didn't share their health worries with their doctor and only visited their GP when already ill. Men are also poorly informed about their health – a MORI poll showed that only a third of men knew anything about their prostate gland although the death rate from prostate cancer is four times that of cervical cancer and that more than one in three men can expect to suffer some form of prostate disease before the age of 50.

'Ask a man how he feels and he will almost invariably say he is fine, regardless of how severely or for how long he has been suffering from a health problem,' says Steve Carroll. 'It is often not until a crisis has occurred and he is on his way to hospital that the true state of his health becomes known.' The message is clear – don't wait for that heart attack. Find someone to talk to about your health and your sexuality – early treatment can not only improve the quality of your life, but sometimes actually save your life too.

Is psychosexual counselling for you?

Therapy is one form of treatment recommended for both men and women, and is often very helpful, though it doesn't appeal to everyone. It may help difficulties with an obvious psychological base, either on its own or in combination with other treatments. Psychosexual counselling may also be effective in dealing with the following circumstances.

- Clearing up emotional problems caused by sexual difficulties with a physical cause. It is by no means uncommon for people to experience a vicious cycle of fear and inadequacy following poor performance which has a phsyical basis, and to experience ongoing difficulties due to a combination of phsyical and psychological causes.
- Helping couples who are trying to re-establish a sexual relationship after a long period of enforced abstinence, after physical treatment has taken place.
- Dealing with underlying emotional issues which may have led to sexual difficulties, as well as the anxiety and fear which may directly prevent sexual activity.

Therapy in a broader sense may be very useful in dealing with 'whole person' issues even if you don't particularly wish to discuss your sexual progress.

FIVE QUICK WAYS TO KEEP POSITIVE

POSITIVE THOUGHTS can impact on our psychological and physical health, and are especially important for improving performance, an area where confidence is key. Good self-esteem can help provide the motivation to tackle potential health problems, such as obesity, as well as enhancing sexuality almost beyond any other measure.

- ***Take some exercise***. It improves the fitness you need for good lovemaking, boosts vitality and improves circulation. Good blood flow, as already explained, is needed for sexual arousal and erection.
- ***Wear bright, alive colours such as green, pink or orange***. These have been shown to be calming, uplifting and warming. They can also improve your confidence, which can be vital for sexual encounters.
- ***Have a healthy snack***. Choose snacks such as honey-sweetened ginger tea and a grated carrot and orange salad to boost your energy and keep your blood sugar level steady so you can't give that 'I'm too tired' excuse.
- ***Listen hard to your inner voice and take action accordingly***. If you are in tune with yourself you will naturally feel more positive and more sure about how to interact with others.
- ***Talk to someone – and listen***. Keeping the flow of sympathy alive between people helps break a depressed mood and makes it easier to reach out, sexually and otherwise.

Sleep

No one feels like making love when groggy and irritable from lack of sleep, yet insomnia and broken nights are suprisingly common, affecting as many as a third of all men and women. Sleep is generally key for good health and effective performance. It helps produce growth hormone which in adults is important for cell repair and renewal. Enough sleep can also keep blood pressure levels normal, according to research at the University of Pavia, Italy. Sleep can help boost your defences against infection, according to research at the University of California at San Diego, which showed that after missing five hours of sleep, people produce fewer of the white blood cells which strengthen the immune system. And sex itself releases endorphins which can result in calm, restful sleep.

There has always been a certain amount of mystique attached to the bed itself. In the mid-18th century in London one John Graham made a fortune charging people for the privilege of sleeping on his 'celestial bed'. The bed was decorated with luxurious hangings, soft music played, scented incense burned and coloured lights played on the sleeper. For his efforts, Graham earned the epithet OWL – Oh Wonderful Love! Without going to these extremes, it does pay to make sure that your bed is how you want it – warm, comfortable and a reflection of your personality, whether you run to a dozen lacy pillows, a four-poster complete with curtains or a minimal futon.

The same applies to the bedroom, the ultimate place of refuge and intimacy, and a place where ideally you feel secure and relaxed enough for lovemaking (though of course this isn't limited to the one location). Keep work and bedroom areas separate and don't take work-related material into the bedroom. Go through the room and de-clutter it – throw out everything you at heart dislike, or haven't worn or used. Get rid of tired old ornaments and buy just one or two pictures or hangings which really mean something to you, and add items which you really like, either fantastical objects such as a four-poster complete with hanging curtains, or something more prosaic like a shower.

TIPS FOR A GOOD NIGHT'S SLEEP

- Sleep should be viewed as part of your whole life, according to healer Deepak Chopra. Sleep or lack of it is closely related to what goes on during your day, so that, for example, unfinished goals, stress and other frustrations can keep you awake, 'churning' for hours. So, decide to tackle unfinished (or unstarted) business by day as much as possible. You may not get it all done in one day, but simply making a start will probably leave you soothed. This applies as much to long-term goals as to day-by-day sources of stress and anxiety. These will obviously take longer to tackle but if ignored may continue to keep you awake until you give them the attention they are demanding.
- Native Americans and Australian aboriginal natives believe in sharing and acting out dreams to release emotional and creative energy. Keep a dream diary – just writing down dreams can help give them shape and meaning. Or, keep a dream diary with a friend or partner on a regular basis, or start a dream-sharing group to help share your dreams further. Sometimes, a succession of disturbing dreams can also disturb sleep, waking you up sporadically throughout the night, or waking you up altogether and leaving you with your mind racing, unable to drop off again. Very disturbing dreams can also leave the person afraid to go back to sleep again. Finding a way of 'unloading' these dreams helps establish the

peaceful mind so needed for good, restful sleep.

- Insomnia can sometimes have a link with the lack of certain nutrients and has been particularly associated with lack of vitamin B6, vitamin C, magnesium and calcium. Too much alcohol, nicotine, and caffeine will also keep you awake.
- Take some exercise during the day, but avoid hard exercise shortly before bed as this will raise your adrenalin levels and leave you too wired to sleep. According to a study in the *European Journal of Applied Physiology*, nine weeks of exercising for 20 minutes three times a week will improve sleep patterns.
- Have a regular wind-down routine around the same time each night – for example, have a bath, read a book or tidy the room.
- Sprinkle a few drops of a soothing oil on your pillow, or use it in a base or carrier oil to massage your partner. Try lavender, rose or camomile, all famous for relieving tension and helping you relax.
- Homeopathic remedies for insomnia include coffea, pulsatilla, rhus tox, arsenicum, nux vomica, silicea, aconite, argentum nit, onosmodium and sepia.
- Herbal remedies include valerian, hops and passionflower.
- Try a simple hydrotherapy technique which is designed to reduce blood flow to the head and help the over-active brain switch off naturally. Place each wrist under a flow of cold water for one minute until your wrists feel cooled but not chilled. Mop your hands, go back to bed and relax, tucking your hands under your arms. Almost immediately, you will be aware of increasing warmth in your hands. While this is happening, the blood supply to your brain is being reduced and the chances are by the time your hands have fully warmed up you may already be nodding off. (For more on the power of water see page 139.)

SPACE AND INTIMACY

KEEPING THE RIGHT balance between being alone and being with someone can sometimes be difficult and indeed can be a major source of stress. Contrary to common belief, a successful sex life does not depend on unbroken intimacy. We all need space sometimes to recharge our batteries and clarify our thinking.

- *Learn to switch off from others*. Don't let your life be overrun by everyone else's needs while you neglect your own.
- *Learn to state clearly when you need to be alone*. Respect your own need for privacy and others will follow suit.
- *Create a sanctuary*. This can be either physical, in terms of a room or space which is just yours, or mental, in terms of a meditation exercise which creates an inner space which is just yours, such as visualizing a walled garden or a remote tropical island.
- *Write down lists of your goals*. Include both long- and short-term goals, to keep your personal Identity and needs alive and strong.
- *Visualize the achievement of these goals*. Visualize this in as much detail as possible – the type of life you will live, how you'll feel, what else you'll be able to do and so on.
- *Go out alone sometimes and try and find different, enjoyable activities*. The stimulation will help feed your current relationship. Physical and emotional enjoyment helps build up your immune system, according to recent research headed by Professor David Warburton, head of psychopharmacology at Reading University. His research showed that happy events seem to build up the body's production of the antibody sigA (secretory Immunoglobin-A), which helps protect against infection and boosts health, so paving the way for a healthy life.

Sensual scents

Appeal in scent is of course largely a matter of personal opinion – what turns one person on may make another feel positively nauseous. However, some scents are said to produce particular effects. Ylang ylang, sandalwood, black pepper, cedarwood, clary sage, fennel, frankincense, ginger, jasmine and rose are just some of the scents supposed to heighten the sensitivity of the erogenous zones and increase receptivity to matters sensual. They can be used in a number of ways – dropped into an oil burner to scent a room, added to a bath, or blended with a base oil such as almond for massage.

Passion-killers – obesity, constipation, bad hygiene and bad breath

There are some problems which effortlessly militate against happy sexual expression, but they can be tackled. The common concept of large people being happy may extend to images of them happily frolicking around on the bed and if this is you, fine; but for others obesity bears specific sexual as well as general health problems. Constipation has perhaps little-known links with low libido, while lack of personal hygiene spoils sexual relations surprisingly often, even if offenders might not like to think so!

OBESITY

Obesity is specifically linked with lower libido, lower sperm count and subfertility. Over the past couple of decades the number of people who are obese or overweight has almost tripled, with one in three people classed as overweight and one in five obese. The general trend to eat more convenience foods affects men especially, who also risk fatigue, poor nutrition and lowered sex drive if they get a lot of their calories from alcohol. Research indicates that one out of 50 males gets nearly a third of his daily energy from alcohol.

The health risks associated with being overweight start when you are as little as 7lb (3.2kg) overweight. Being overweight is particularly linked with circulatory diseases such as angina, atherosclerosis or

Pheromones

PHEROMONES ARE COMPLEX chemical substances which are released by most female mammals around ovulation, and which have the effect of attracting a mate at the time when pregnancy (and the continuation of the species) is most likely to result. This is an aspect of the biological or 'selfish gene' theory, which says that we are genetically programmed for maximum reproduction. Interestingly, research shows that women wear shorter skirts when ovulating.

With regard to pheromones, women secrete organic acids such as acetic acid and butanic acid around ovulation, which according to John Mann, author and professor of organic chemistry at Reading University, could best be described as a mixture of vinegar and rancid butter! Also, male sweat contains breakdown products of testosterone which in concentrated form smell of urine. In trace amounts, both chemicals have a musky odour and may act as aphrodisiacs, says Professor Mann. However, due to modern hygiene, many people's output of pheromones is often too low or is covered up.

DID YOU KNOW? Celery contains pheromones and is reputed to be an aphrodisiac – or is it just the phallic shape? For more on aphrodisiacs, see Chapter 3; tips on sexy nutrients can be found in Chapter 4.

hardening of the arteries, stroke, hypertension or high blood pressure, heart attack, poor circulation and varicose veins. Given the importance of good blood flow for successful erection, these all have obvious relevance, apart of course from people's natural desire to stay alive. Diabetes is another risk of being overweight, which again is a common cause of loss of sexual desire.

And, though some people delight in having a partner of size, for others this is not the case. Being overweight may erode self-confidence and may not be not conducive to attracting a partner. Food can also be a psychological comforter which some people turn to when their sensuality isn't released in other ways – it can be quite easy to get into the habit of eating together instead of making love together. However, on the positive side, habits can always be reversed.

Tackling the problem

- *Aim to build weight loss into your overall lifestyle in gradual easy stages.* That way, it's most likely to last. Try and think in terms of healthy eating – dieting is old-fashioned and usually ineffective. And try and enjoy yourself and your partner as you are now – don't wait to attain that perfect weight.
- *Set realistic targets.* Don't try and lose the accumulated weight of months or years in a week. Aim to lose 1–2lb (0.5–1kg) a week *maximum* over an initial period of a month. Then reassess the situation and try it for another month. Keeping your goals short-term helps keep you optimistic and motivated. If you try and diet more quickly, you may lose muscle instead of fat, and your metabolism can slow by up to 30 per cent, making you more likely to regain lost weight and more once you start eating again.
- *Don't be discouraged by binges.* Pick up the pieces and go on eating sensibly – but do try and analyse why you binged. What emotional

factors make you eat? Is it frustration, boredom, a relationship, work? Eating is a very short-term way of dealing with problems, so make an effort to set aside time to create deeper resolutions.

- *Break the habit.* Keep busy at times when you're most likely to eat without being hungry, commonly the evening. Join a dating agency or a charity which needs volunteer help, for example.
- *Be a disciplined shopper.* Don't go shopping when you're hungry. Make a list and stick to it. Having a budget can be helpful – take a set amount in cash so you're not tempted to splash out on fattening foods such as chocolate biscuits.
- *Change your eating habits.* Simple changes in eating habits can help the weight fall off (so if you haven't done so already, read the opening part of this chapter which deals with healthy eating).
- *Have a test for food allergies.* Some people also lose weight and retained water when they discover and tackle food allergies and intolerances. Common foods and drinks can be enough to cause tiredness, depression and loss of interest in sex, including coffee, sugar, wheat and dairy products.
- *Allow yourself and your partner some sensual snacks.* Try oysters and champagne in bed by candlelight, for example. The sequel may distract you from having a second course!

CONSTIPATION

Constipation, definitely unsexy as it is, has been linked with low libido. The rectum and sex organs are linked by branches of the same nerve, and, on a psychological basis, sometimes 'holding back' in one area can be mirrored by similar restraint in the other. It's much better to improve your diet than to go for laxatives, which can cause harm by washing valuable nutrients out of the body.

Tackling the problem

To deal with severe constipation in the first instance, try a few dried figs soaked in water with a little honey and two or three teaspoons of linseed (available from health food shops and pharmacists). Other remedies include prunes or plums, pineapple juice, apples, and other fruit.

On a more regular basis, to prevent constipation:

- *Drink four or five glasses of water a day.* Drink it plain, with half a squeezed lemon or lime, as herbal teas, or mixed with natural fruit juice.
- *Eat healthy foods.* Include lots of fresh fruit and vegetables in your diet, as well as fibre-rich foods such as oats, wholegrain bread, brown rice. Natural 'live' yoghurt also helps keep your digestive tract healthy.
- *Improve your diet in general.* Some forms of constipation are linked with nutrient deficiencies, such as calcium, magnesium and vitamin B6.
- *Get regular exercise.*

GENERAL HYGIENE

General hygiene rules are obvious but sometimes neglected, for example when a person lacks the energy to take a shower or bath, or sometimes through sheer lack of awareness. A daily routine of hygiene can go beyond cleanliness, vital though this is, it is refreshing, energizing and can also increase awareness. The close attention you give your body during washing, showering or bathing gives you a closer knowledge of it, which in turn gives you the power to create better health by changing anything which needs to be changed. To take a very basic example, taking a bath or shower is the time when you're most likely to notice anything amiss with the sexual organs such as a rash, lump or wart.

KISS BAD BREATH GOODBYE

Sexual confidence and performance can all too easily be blown away by bad breath. A whiff of foul air from someone else's mouth is an effective turn-off, while individuals who suspect they have bad breath can find it an absolutely debilitating problem.

Causes of bad breath

Halitosis is often caused by bacteria in the mouth but there are various specific causes which can be tackled.

- *'Morning breath'*. We probably all have some degree of this. Normally the mouth self-cleans by the flow of saliva, rich in oxygen, which naturally slows down during the night. Normal tooth brushing deals with this, as does breakfast, which starts the saliva flowing again. Flossing also helps.
- *Dry mouth*. Anything which dries up the normal cleansing flow of saliva may cause bad breath, such as breathing through the mouth, alcohol, hunger or even too much talking! Stress can also cause bad breath, though it isn't known why. One woman apparently developed bad breath whenever her boyfriend made sexual advances! Perhaps it is something to do with the way breathing patterns change under stress. Drinking more liquid may help, as may sugar-free chewing gum, which improves the flow of saliva.
- *Gum disease*. Periodontal disease is the classic cause of persistent bad breath, as plaque may form a seal over gums and teeth which blocks out oxygen, so creating the perfect environment for bacteria. Your dentist can prescribe a course of antibiotics or antifungal medication.
- *Sulphur-producing bacteria*. These are another cause of bad breath, especially at the back of the tongue. Brushing the tongue regularly

can root out these bacteria. Your tongue is clean if it's a healthy pink.

- *Dentures.* Dentures can cause problems, especially if they fit poorly, and need scrupulous cleaning.
- *Cigarettes.* Tobacco has been noted as a cause of halitosis for centuries. King James VI, writing his *Counterblast to Tobacco* in 1604, remarked, 'Herein is a great contempt, that the sweetnesse of man's breath, being a good gift of God, should be wilfully corrupted by this stinking smoke.' The great cure for this one is giving up.
- *Booze.* Alcohol causes a temporary taint on the breath, and can also dry up the saliva needed to sweeten your breath.
- *Garlic.* Powerful as a breath tainter, the only cure is the passage of time.
- *Dieting.* This can cause a dry mouth. Also, when dieters burn off their fat stores it gives off acetone, which has a medicinal smell. Make sure you clean your mouth and tongue and drink plenty of water and juice.
- *Illness.* Some medical conditions can produce bad breath as a symptom. Sinusitis for example can produce bad breath because a person is forced to breathe through the mouth, so causing dry mouth, and also because some sinus infections are caused by bacteria which produce sulphur gases. Other conditions which can cause bad breath include tonsillitis, throat infections, hiatus hernia, diabetes, kidney failure and liver failure. Some women also find they get bad breath just before a period, thought to be due to hormonal imbalance.

CHAPTER FOUR

Alternative or Complementary Therapies

Sexuality more obviously than many issues is a whole person concern, occupying a sometimes inflammable area between the physical, emotional and spiritual. One of the deepest form of communication between individuals, it is also an arena where social truths are played out, and is a litmus test of health in its broadest sense. If we have trouble defining health in a general sense, describing good sexual health is even more elusive. Sexual health as absence of symptoms is almost meaningless, though any adverse symptoms in this area do need medical investigation. Optimum terms are needed in describing peak sexual health – a sense of joy, liberation, and supreme ease both of body and mind. With sex perhaps even more than health conditions, a holistic approach is needed which takes into account inner as well as outer factors, and which interprets sexuality in a larger context than the health of the genitals or even the health of the body.

Alternative and complementary remedies form the ideal meeting place for this holistic approach. Here, sex can be as physical or as mental or as spiritual as you like. You choose the balance, without it being imposed on you by outside factors. In this often sensitive area, it is entirely up to you how much or how little you reveal, and which areas you choose to work upon, and there are many alternative therapies, offering a vast choice of directions. Whether you want to boost your general energy level, deal with specific sexual difficulties, become fitter or find and maintain deep inner equilibrium you should be able to find a complementary therapy to suit your needs.

Many complementary therapies are grounded in ancient disciplines which have known about sexual problems for a long time, and have evolved sophisticated and precise ways of treating them. These therapies may work on several levels. Some work directly on sexual energy, perhaps by balancing hormones or improving blood flow, while others work indirectly on the cause of sexual problems in various ways, depending what the causes are. Other therapies work more generally and aim at boosting energy and reviving the body. Still other therapies may be off-beat and offer highly individual routes to increased sexual awareness. Natural therapies can also be used to expand awareness and further spiritual development, on the premise that the more developed the individual consciousness, the richer relationships are likely to be. Last but by no means least, undertaking them is often fun, which in itself can be very effective in releasing tension and creating a positive, confident mood for intimacy.

There is no doubt that alternative medicine is here to stay, reflecting the growing responsibility we are taking for our own health. Two in five Americans use alternative medicine, according to a report published in the *Journal of the American Medical Association*. The thousand people surveyed said it wasn't because they were 'fed up with conventional medicine' but because they view health more holistically. Visits to alternative medicine practitioners have increased by almost 50 per cent over the past decade and exceeded the visits to all US primary-care physicians.

Sex can often be an area for guilt, but attending to your personal needs in this area, is more likely to lead to a healthy outcome than ignoring or suppressing them. The process can sometimes be invigorating and rejuvenating, occasionally painful. Ultimately, it is grounded in the willingness to explore, sometimes to take risks or let go, and become involved in life. It is this questing attitude, this zest for adventure, which can so enrich your quality of life, sexual and otherwise.

This chapter looks at alternative techniques which may be useful both for flagging desire and outright sexual dysfunction in both men and women. Many of the remedies can be started at home, though some will need professional supervision by an expert should you wish to take them further. The therapies are listed in alphabetical order.

The Alexander Technique

The Alexander Technique aims to teach you how to hold your body and move more correctly. Its founder Frederick Matthias Alexander, an actor working in the 1920s, believed that many of us unwittingly learn bad habits of posture and movement which then affect our health, mood and general wellbeing, which can be un-learned using the Alexander Technique. For example, the technique aims to re-align the head so that it sits correctly in line with the spine, which in turn impacts positively on a person's entire energy and wellbeing. Using the Alexander Technique can help us to understand how the body is naturally designed to work, and can heighten awareness on many levels. It aims to teach – or re-educate – us how to use the body in such a way as to maximize psychological balance along with physical efficiency. It may help you get in touch with your body and its needs generally, and to release any

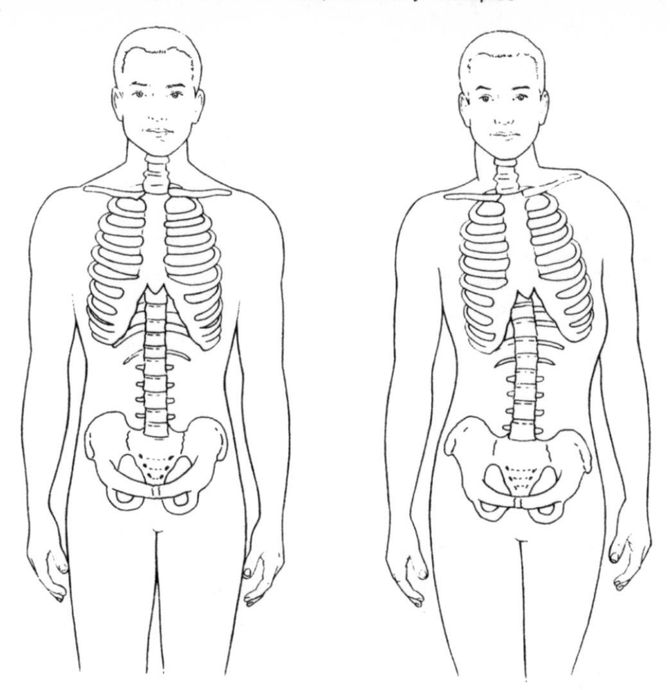

1 Unbalanced posture, above, can put a strain on the entire skeletal system, as well as the internal organs, affecting a person's energy and wellbeing.

tension which has been blocking sexual expression. While the Alexander Technique is not a sexual therapy as such, it may well activate the body's natural self-healing mechanisms, helping raise low energy levels and overcome minor ailments which can result in low libido.

American studies indicate that the Alexander Technique can improve breathing and appears to lengthen the neck muscles. An ongoing study at Kingston Hospital, London, indicates it can help relieve chronic back pain, which is a surprisingly common cause of sexual problems as described in Chapter 3. Certainly, many doctors now recommend the Alexander Technique for poor posture, stress and pain.

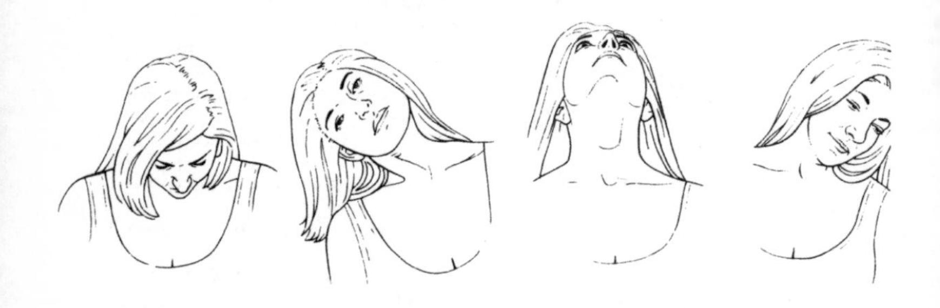

2 Head roll.

Ideally, you should attend a session in person to get the full benefit, as many people have to be physically shown their poor habits – that is, they have to be gently pulled and prodded into place! As a starting point, however, you could try working on your neck area. It may seem a little far removed from the sex organs, but Alexander realized that the root cause of many problems was the over-tightening of the neck muscles which threw the whole body out of balance, down the spine and into the pelvic area. Certainly, releasing tension in this area can help combat the stress which can destroy desire. Alexander recommended three main directions.

1 Allow the neck to be free

This is to get rid of excess tension which is so often found in the neck muscles. You may find a yoga exercise helpful as a starting point (see Figure 2: Head roll) though it is recommended you attend a class where you can be instructed in person.

2 Allow the head to go forward and upward

This helps the mechanisms of the body to function naturally and freely. The head is balanced in such a way that, when the neck muscles are released, the head goes slightly forward, which takes the whole body into movement. The way to do this is to allow the head to go forward as if you were about to nod in agreement. Again, personal supervision is recommended in order to learn the technique properly.

3 Allow the back to lengthen and widen

Since the spine shortens because of excess muscular tension when the head is pulled back, allowing the back to lengthen may actually raise your height. This can be encouraged by imagining that a string attached to the top of your head is pulling you up towards the ceiling.

Art therapy

Art therapy can help people express their feelings very vividly and accurately without words and can be a powerful tool for the release of emotions. First used after World War II with shell-shocked soldiers and home-coming prisoners of war, and thereafter a feature of psychiatric treatment, art therapy is now increasingly used for relationship difficulties, or to boost self-esteem. Art therapy can also be used to portray conflicts about sexuality, or emotions around a potentially sexually limiting condition such as poor circulation, diabetes or epilepsy.

Some therapists offer a mix of art therapy and counselling for both individuals and couples. At St Luke's Hospital in the UK, a counselling session is followed by the couple drawing a picture of their view of their

The power of colour

IF YOU DRAPE yourself and/or your lover in a rich shade of red to raise the passion level, will it work?

The use of colour to change mood and health has a long history. Seven primary wavelengths or vibrations of colour have had healing and mystical significance since ancient times. The colours of the spectrum visible to the human eye – red, orange, yellow, green, blue, indigo and violet – were believed to have specific effects on the human body by many former civilizations including the ancient Indians, Chinese, Tibetans, Egyptians, Greeks, Persians and Babylonians. Healing with colour has been in use for thousands of years in China and in India, where it forms part of the Ayurvedic medical tradition.

Red, the colour with the longest visible wavelength, is associated with the body and with sexual and other passions, the mind with yellow, and the spirit with blue. Followers of Pythagoras believed that the seven colours of the spectrum corresponded to the eight notes of the scale, with both the first and eighth notes corresponding to red (the eighth having a higher vibration of red).

Colour therapy takes different forms, including colour breathing, which comprises visualizing coloured breath being inhaled and exhaled during meditation. (For more on breathing therapies generally, see the section on Breathwork on page 104.) Colour therapy also includes being exposed to coloured lights or materials, eating certain coloured foods or drinking water steeped in sunlight in coloured containers. Colours may have specific therapeutic uses – blue may be used to treat high blood pressure, insomnia or stress, for example. Some scientific research suggests that colour may affect the body, in that the perception of colour by the eye seems to trigger biochemical reactions. However, the greatest effect is likely to be on mood. In aura healing, practitioners visualize healing colours to heal the aura, said to be made up of colours of its own.

relationship now, and another showing how they would like it to be. The drawings, which should not be shown to their partner, are then analysed at the next session and can provide a fruitful starting point for discussion.

The use of colour in particular forms almost a whole separate language. Dark, drab colours have obvious significance, as may the passionate or angry shade of red. Blue has connotations of coldness, black of sadness or endings and green of growth. Although many people in art therapy may use colour without being consciously aware of the significance of the colour shades, the therapeutic use of colour goes back a very long way into the collective psyche (see box).

Ayurveda

Ayurveda, the ancient Indian art of healing, was introduced in Chapter 2, which looked at herbal and other remedies for impotence and low desire. Ayurveda is a Sanskrit word meaning 'the science of life and longevity'. According to Ayurveda, every person is a creation of cosmic energies, with a unique personality and constitution which is our individual psychobiological makeup. People are said to belong to one of three energy types, or *doshas*, and depending on which type you are, and your individual needs, an Ayurvedic practitioner will prescribe a mix of remedies designed to restore and maintain the body's equilibrium.

MASSAGE

For impotence and low libido, Ayurveda includes several massage options, not with the aim of stimulating sexually, but either to improve circulation or to boost the body's energy.

Massage for impotence

Massage can be a useful treatment in cases of impotence as it can improve circulation and a good blood flow is essential to erection. Specific remedies for impotence suggested by Ayurvedic expert Dr Vasant Lad include the following.

- Massaging the pubic area (the lower part of the abdomen) and the root of the penis with a few drops of *mahanarayan* oil, which will improve circulation and may be enough to solve the problem. *Bala* oil or *ashwagandha* oil can also be applied directly to the penis; or, if you don't have these oils, ghee will do (see page 103).
- Massaging over the prostate gland, halfway between the scrotum and anus.
- A massage for low libido is to gently press the head of the penis (the glans penis) with the top of the index finger, aiming for the groove about one inch behind the tip of the penis. A *marma* point is located at the centre of that groove which in Ayurvedic terms means that it is an energy point on the skin which is connected to the inner pathways of healing.

DIET

There are several strengthening dietary remedies for both men and women with low libido that you can try for yourself. They are all recommended by Dr Lad as being effective at restoring sexual energy.

- *Raw almond drink.* Soak 10 raw almonds overnight, peel and blend with 1 cup warm milk, 1 teaspoon ghee, 1 teaspoon natural sugar, a pinch of nutmeg and saffron.
- *Fresh dates.* Soak 10 fresh dates in a quart of ghee, then add

1 teaspoon ginger, a tiny pinch of cardamom, and a pinch of saffron. Cover and place in a warm place for at least two weeks. Then eat one date a day in the early morning.

- *Figs and honey.* After breakfast, eat three figs with one teaspoon of honey. An hour later, drink a glass of lassi. (To make lassi, blend one tablespoon of fresh yoghurt with one cup of water and a pinch of cumin powder.)
- *Garlic milk.* Mix together one cup of milk, a quarter cup of water, and one clove of garlic. Simmer until only one cup of liquid remains and drink at bedtime. It may also be helpful to add more garlic and onions to your diet.

To make ghee

Put 2lb/1kg unsalted butter into a heavy saucepan and heat gently until it melts, being careful not to burn the butter. Simmer very gently for 12–15 minutes until the ghee is golden and forms whitish curds. When the curds turn a light tan, take it off the heat at once and allow to cool until the ghee is just warm and the curds have settled to the bottom. Decant the ghee into a container and discard the curds. It will keep without refrigeration.

Ghee is said to have several medicinal properties, such as lubricating the body's connective tissue and so making the body more flexible. It can also can be used for massage as described above. However – which may be relevant for men with impotence – ghee should be used with caution by those with high cholesterol, and also by both men and women who are overweight.

These massage and diet remedies can obviously easily be tried at home, but if you decide to consult an Ayurvedic practitioner, you will receive a much more holistic approach. As already explained in Chapter 2, impotence and low desire are viewed within the context of the overall situation. Generally, however, (as with other medical disciplines) impotence is viewed as often having an underlying physical cause, such as thickening of the arteries. In Ayurvedic terms, low libido is viewed as a symptom indicating that overall body energy is lacking, and an Ayurvedic practitioner will look at different ways to boost it, including diet, lifestyle, exercise, rest and relaxation as well as additional therapies such as sound, colour and aromatherapy if necessary. You may want to consult a practitioner if you feel your problems won't respond to simple self-help measures, or if you want a thorough, overall investigation.

Breathwork

Breathwork is the name for a variety of breathing techniques which can be used consciously to work with our most vital unconscious biological function, breathing. It is well known how energy and inner calm can be increased with yoga breathing, or *pranayama*, which draws in the life energy or *prana*, and breathing techniques have been used in India for centuries as a means of raising physical, mental and spiritual awareness. In China, breathing exercises form an important part of tai chi (see page 132). Eastern cultures believe correct breathing is necessary for physical and spiritual health and that we take in life-enhancing energy or prana every time we inhale. Poor breathing is believed to contribute to a range of problems including high blood pressure, fatigue, insomnia and depression, all of which can contribute to poor sexual performance.

The most common fault as regards breathing is that we tend to breathe too shallowly, in which case it can be easy to lose the rhythm of lovemaking, or even to panic – a reaction which can effectively terminate sex. Breath needs to be taken right into the depths of the body for maximum renewal and the calmness needed to carry sexual encounters through.

Breathwork includes modern breathing techniques such as Holotropic Breathwork (see box), Circle Breathing and Transformational Breathing. Some therapists believe that past trauma or current tension damage the natural breathing pattern and become ingrained in people's breathing habits, so contributing to stress and health problems. They will use relaxing breathing techniques to reach a primal repose in which healing can take place, and good breathing habits taught. This kind of therapy may be useful if you have become emotionally tangled about making

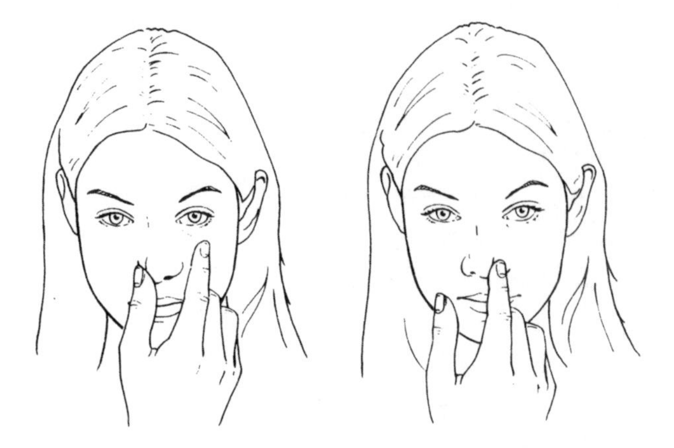

3 Close your right nostril with your right thumb and inhale through your left nostril. Hold for a few seconds, then exhale through your right nostril, closing the left nostril with the ring finger of your right hand. Now inhale through the right nostril; hold, and exhale through the left nostril. Repeat for a minute or two.

love, either because of old psychological trauma, or simply because physical difficulties mean you have lost confidence and need a little help to get back on track.

HOLOTROPIC BREATHWORK

HOLOTROPIC BREATHWORK (holotropic means 'moving towards wholeness') was developed by Dr Stanislov Grof, a psychiatrist, and by Christina Grof, a transpersonal teacher. Based on a melange of modern consciousness research, depth psychology and established spiritual practices, holotropic breathwork aims to create altered states of consciousness which activate an individual's spontaneous healing potential. This may be especially helpful for lowered libido due to stress or psychological factors, though some practitioners believe it may also have a releasing effect on physical traumas which have become trapped in the body, so blocking sexual expression. Sustained effective breathing, evocative music, focused energy work, and mandala drawing, all form part of this form of breathwork.

BREATHING TIPS

- Before making love, take three yoga deep breaths to combat stress and maximize energy. Inhale deeply from the abdomen to a count of ten, hold for a moment, then exhale to a count of ten.
- If you feel tired and apathetic about making love, try six to eight short inhalations straight into the belly to give the body a quick energy charge.
- Alternate nostril breathing (see Figure 3) is sometimes said to balance male and female energies in Ayurvedic or yogic terms. It is also said to charge the two halves of the brain, so leading to overall neurological and physical balance and raising the energy needed for sexual encounters.

Chanting

As well as rhythmical breathing techniques, shamans and native medicine men use chanting as an innate part of sexuality, initiation and fertility rites. Chanting is used as part of tribal society rituals to obtain an altered state of consciousness to help heal problems such as sexual dysfunction, to lift libido, and generally to raise consciousnes of sexual prowess and potential. The Navajo chant elaborate myths as part of curing rituals which also include sand painting. The long texts must be chanted perfectly otherwise not only are they ineffective, but counterproductive, resulting in the condition they were supposed to cure. Some Navajo still will not accept conventional medical treatment without an accompanying 'chantway'.

The most common methods involve chanting 'power songs' which cause a change in breathing patterns on the path to inward 'travelling'. Words vary from individual to individual, but melodies and rhythms are handed down from generation to generation, and are likely to include specific ones for matters sexual.

Chanting is also traditionally used by groups to raise a communal psychic field of energy, a tradition which persists among modern witches, or adherents of the Craft, and Pagans (and also, to a less conscious extent, among Christians who sing hymns in church). Witches combine chanting and dancing to raise a 'cone of power' which is then released to work a spell or create healing. If required, the power released could be channelled towards healing sexual disorders. The chants may be names of goddesses or the horned god, or phrases from spells. Psychic witches can sometimes see the cone as a luminous cloud or a silver-blue light. In magic, the success of a spell is also said to depend heavily on the sound vibrations created by chanting, a belief which dates back thousands of years. The ancient Egyptians were aware of the power of sound upon people, a belief which still underlies modern sound therapy or sound healing today, which often makes use of native American, Tibetan or Mongolian chants.

Soundings: The Shamanic journey

PRESENT-DAY SHAMANS, drawing on psychophysical practices which date back some 35,000 years, use chanting and other sound work to achieve an altered state of consciousness which some believe may underly the practice for which shamans are traditionally most famous – the sensation of flying.

Soundwork may be undertaken for the sake of the 'journey' itself – the adventure of exploring and extending the mind beyond its usual limits – or as a form of deep meditation, on the premise that normal consciousness may be too limited to find creative solutions to problems. Sexuality is also viewed by some as encompassing an altered state of consciousness, so that shamanic work may help explore this aspect of consciousness with beneficial effect on sexual expression.

Drums, rattles and tapes as well as chanting all form part of shamanistic soundwork, along with any 'helper applications' such as fasting, incense, candles, working in darkness or facing the sun though these are not regarded as essential and should only be used if you really find them useful. As with other forms of meditation, some shamanistic soundwork involves listening to the sound, and to the silence which underlies it. As a result, you may achieve mystical inspiration, including insights into your own sexuality, or a state of deep relaxation and balance from which you return refreshed.

Sound therapy aims to expand consciousness, empower and relax, and so could be useful for getting in touch with sexual areas of yourself which you feel you may have lost, for example, if you have been enforcedly celibate for a long time and want to resume sexual relations, or if you need to come to terms with areas of sexual conflict. This kind of therapy can also be confidence-boosting and can be combined with physical treatments for physical causes of sexual dysfunction, such as Shiatsu (see page 126).

Flotation

Flotation simply involves floating effortlessly in water. Widely used to induce deep relaxation, part of flotation's appeal may well go back to foetal memories of the weightless safety of the womb. The therapeutic effects of deep relaxation via flotation may be general, giving a general boost to the system, or helping strengthen the immune system. Flotation has also been used more specifically to counteract stress (research indicates it may help reduce production of adrenalin, the stress hormone), high blood pressure, migraines and back pain. It has also been recommended for low libido, and may be useful for those whose lack of desire is caused by stress, or who suffer erectile dysfunction stemming from poor blood flow.

Flotation therapy developed in the fifties from the work of Dr John Lilly, an American neurophysiologist and psychoanalyst, who devised sensory deprivation chambers as a way of finding out how the brain reacted when denied external stimulus. It involves lying in a sound-proofed, completely dark, tank of warm water which effectively blocks off the outside world completely. The water, comfortably warm, contains enough salt and minerals for the body to float effortlessly. If you're worried you may get panicky or claustrophobic, you can switch on a light or open the door any time.

If you prefer, you may find some of the hydrotherapy treatments suggested on pages 139–141 easier to do at home.

Healing

'Healing' does not mean 'curing'. It deals more with the transfer of energy from healer to patient, a transaction which may involve a psychological shedding of burdens, and feeling more spiritually balanced. Healers believe they channel energy to the patient through the laying on of hands, or at a distance through the power of thought or prayer. Healers work in different ways, including laying on of hands, distance healing, and deep psychological work and others, to identify and remove any negativity which could be blocking health and happiness.

Healing may involve positive experiences of peace and wellbeing, but it may also sometimes be uncomfortable if the therapist is shifting blocked energy. The hands of healers often have a sudden surge of warmth when the healing process is taking place, a warmth which may also be communicated to the patient.

Some doctors now refer patients to healers, or have healers as visiting or regular members of staff. In the UK, reputable healers may not promise miracle cures, and may be members of the National Federation of Spiritual Healers. Healing may in particular help with stress, anxiety and high blood pressure, as well as psychological and emotional blocks which could be blocking full sexual expression.

There are many different types of healing. Two popular ones are therapeutic touch and Reiki. Therapuetic touch involves a form of healing in which practitioners believe the body has unique energy fields and use their hands to rebalance disruptions in the energy flow. Reiki is a form of Japanese healing which practitioners claim causes the body's molecules to vibrate with higher intensity, so dissolving energy blockages.

Human Design

Many astrologers use computers to plot a character analysis which can be useful in choosing a partner or understanding why your lovelife is as it is. A concept called Human Design originated in New Mexico in the late 80s, and was brought to the UK by Richard Rudd, who claims it goes much deeper than usual readings, being a computer method which offers a blueprint of you and your unique essence. In fact, Human Design is not astrology, or an intuitive reading, but is said to be a clear and simple analysis of your biogenetic inheritance. Used in this way, Human Design does not focus on symptoms or healing, but goes for the root of the problem, which is believed to be how we are living our life. Viewed in this way, impotence and low desire are seen as direct reflections of inappropriate living – in general, to reach a state of impotence is to have strayed in some way from one's true nature.

Before starting to do Human Design analysis, Richard Rudd travelled the world, teaching and practising a healing technique from China called Ch'i Nei Tsang. This works on the 'Hara', which is loosely translated as our 'centre of being'. While doing this work, Richard saw and helped many cases, using a similar approach to the

Human Design one he uses now. 'The basis of it is this: when a person lives according to their true nature, they do not need medicine, ever,' says Richard. 'Even when someone becomes ill (which is a part of life, after all) the illness does not need to be fixed. Human Design, and working with the Hara, are more concerned with guiding people back towards their own true nature. This almost always involves a radical change in the outlook of a person's life', such as a change in career or just in fundamental outlook. According to Richard Rudd, it is not really enough to come for a Human Design reading without then putting into practice what you have heard.

Human Design uses elements from the *I'Ching*, the Chinese Book of Changes, in that the genetic code has the same mathematical alignment as the *I'Ching* – 64 hexagrams, and 64 possible arrangements of codons of the genetic code. (Hexagrams are arrangements of lines which form a special meaning; codons are trios of the chemical bases, or nucleotides, which represent the genetic code or hereditary blueprint of each individual.)

In practice, this computer method will give you two readings, one based on the date of your birth, the other from roughly three months beforehand before when the neo-cortex, and so your subconscious, was being formed and biogenetic information 'downloaded' into the developing brain. The result is a body map of nine centres or zones with circuits which might or might not be triggered into action by a partner depending on who he or she is. This approach, in Human Design terms, might be useful in indicating where a person may have strayed from his or her true nature, usually due to conditioning and pressure from the outside world, so resulting in sexual difficulties.

Laughter therapy

A dose of this is probably essential when considering sexuality, as a good time in bed is not guaranteed by taking sex too seriously! Laughter shakes tension out of the body and helps dispel any stress which may be impairing performance. Again, this could be a good therapy to undertake with a partner, either privately or more consciously through a laughter therapist.

The use of humour to reduce stress and improve health by producing changes in the immune system has been the topic of much research. A study at Indiana State University looked at the effectiveness of humour in moderating the effects of stress on the immune system. Thirty-three women watched a funny video, while subjects in the control group viewed two 'straight' videos. Stress scores decreased significantly more in the humour group than in the control group, and the more people laughed, the greater the decreases in stress tended to be – interesting in view of the links between stress and impaired sexual performance. Merely watching the funny video did not lower stress – 'laughter responses' were needed for this. It is thought that the act of laughing produces physiological responses within the body which result in relaxation and enhanced wellbeing (not unlike the physiological responses to sex). The study concluded that humour can reduce stress and enhance or optimize immune function.

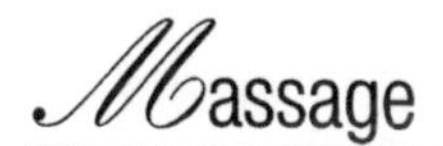

Massage

Massage certainly has sexual connotations, and arousal may be encouraged by a partner massaging erogenous zones, but massage has a far broader application than this and can also be used therapeutically.

Touch is in many ways the oldest sense – it's the sense which develops first in the baby in the womb, and throughout our childhood and adult lives we remain aware of its vital importance to our wellbeing.

The therapeutic benefits of massage can go deeper. Many therapists believe that old trauma from childhood is stored or 'stuck' in the body, and becomes a cellular or biological truth, and that the only way to shift it is by deep massage. Various forms of massage exist which focus on the body's energy points or chakras, and massage can form part of a physical or spiritual healing process depending on which healer you approach.

SELF-MASSAGE

A brisk self-massage can help boost circulation and relax tension, and may be enough to improve blood flow for successful erection or to help with stress-impaired performance. You can perform simple self-massage techniques at home which will bring fresh blood to the tissues, help eliminate waste products, and generally tone up skin and muscles.

The following is a very simple self-massage, working from the neck down to waist level.

- Place a towel behind your neck and, holding either end, pull it from left to right. This creates gentle friction which helps get the circulation moving. You can also do the same with a loofah or natural sponge.
- Place the towel behind your back at the level of the upper arms. Lean back slightly, hands not too far apart, and again pull the towel from left to right.

- Lower the towel again until it is just above waist level. Lean back slightly and pull quite vigorously to the left and then to the right.

AROMATHERAPY

Aromatherapy involves massage with healing herbal oils, the use of which goes back at least 2,000 years. Essential oils as we know them today developed in Persia about a thousand years ago and were brought back to Europe. By the Middle Ages they were popular as medicines and perfumes. Aromatherapy has a big following in France where doctors sometimes prescribe it as an alternative to conventional drugs. However, if you want to use the oils yourself, aromatherapy massage can be done at home by your partner or another friend simply to relax you and help remove negative thoughts, without any onus to perform sexually. Taking away the pressure to perform can sometimes have excellent results!

Used by a professional aromatherapist, this kind of massage aims at relaxing muscle tension and improving circulation – which could obviously be good for erectile dysfunction. It may also be used to heal underlying areas of pain, such as a bad back, or to correct conditions within the body, such as hormonal imbalances. Geranium and rose are two oils often used for balancing female hormones. The aromatherapist might use different oils to reduce stress in a massage which ideally leaves you relaxed but re-energized. Sedative oils include sandalwood, majoram and bergamot; stimulating ones include basil, orange blossom and ylang ylang.

The oils are believed to be absorbed into the body via the skin and are then carried around the body in the bloodstream. Tell your aromatherapist if you are pregnant or if you suffer from epilepsy as certain oils are not recommended in these conditions. Oils may also work through their scents, which are thought to act on the hypothalamus, a part of the brain which influences the hormonal system. We all know how evocative certain scents can be and it is believed that smell is a major part of what attracts the opposite sex and creates arousal (see pheromones, page 88).

Oils do need to be handled with care, so always consult a qualified aromatherapist. If using your oils yourself, make sure they are of good quality, that you follow any instructions on how to use them, and that you are aware of circumstances in which you should not use them.

Effleurage

Different types of massage strokes exist but one which may be especially suitable for aromatherapy is effleurage, which is smooth, gentle and puts no pressure on the body. All the same, effleurage is profound in its effects because of the way it penetrates the skin and feeds back to the brain. It can really help a person get in touch with his or her physical body but without any undue pressure.

To do an aromatherapy massage on the back:

- The person receiving the massage will be lying face down while the person giving the massage should be standing at one side of the head.
- Place your hands lightly on the other person's upper back.
- Keeping your elbows straight, slowly glide down either side of the spine, maintaining an even pressure.
- Sweep your hands up and around the pelvis, then back along the edges of the chest and up to the shoulder. Repeat 20 times.

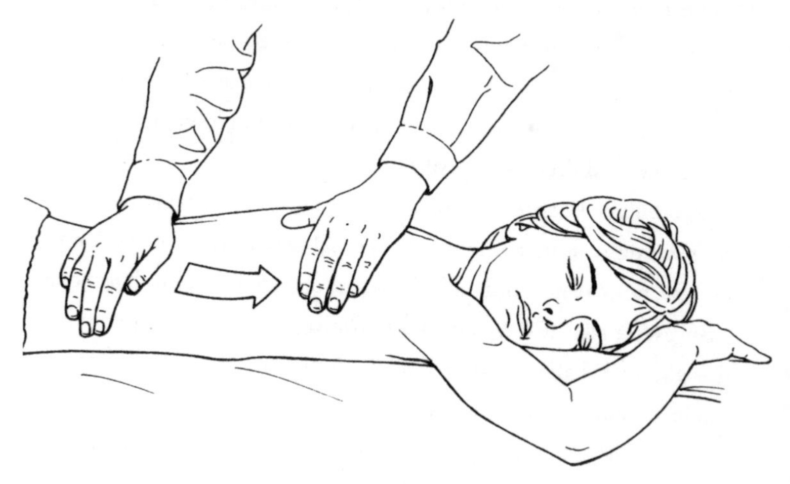

4 An aromatherapy massage.

Meditation (reaching sexual health via the fourth dimension)

It is now widely accepted that the body responds to your state of mental and emotional awareness, but accessing this link can be difficult in our stressed-out culture. Meditation can provide an easy way to tune in if you can bypass the common idea that it involves effort and strain and a relentless blocking out of all external stimuli. One of the easiest and most effective forms of meditation, Transcendental Meditation (TM), simply involves listening to an inner or outer sound, or personal mantra. Adherents of TM say this mantra is best taught personally by a qualified TM teacher to avoid negative effects caused by the improper use of sacred sound. The mind naturally seeks *turiya* or the fourth state (i.e. not waking, sleeping or dreaming). This fourth state of transcendental consciousness goes beyond ordinary experiences, and studies have shown how people who practise it experience changes in metabolism such as lowered blood pressure and heart rate, and decreased oxygen consumption.

According to Deepak Chopra, it in this state of meditation that 'mind over matter' can best help create optimal health. As Chopra points out, the normal state of mind of anyone, including an unwell person, changes from day to day, sometimes positive, sometimes negative, with thoughts at a shallow or deep level. In this vacillating, everyday state, results of 'mind over matter' are likely to be variable and not always effective. TM offers a way to contact what Chopra calls 'the hidden blueprint of intelligence' and change it; in the fourth dimension, Chopra suggests that we are able to 'talk' directly to our DNA, the genetic blueprint of our being. This view posits that the human body is controlled by a 'network of intelligence' grounded in quantum reality in which, ultimately, energy and matter are believed to be interchangeable hence, this intelligence goes deep enough to change the basic physiological patterns which dictate our health. Only then can visualization be strong enough to realize individual desires in terms of peak health and performance.

Naturopathy

Since the 17th century, Western medicine has been based on the Cartesian principle of dualism, or the separation of body and mind. Naturopathy, which simply means natural treatment, is a discipline which aims at holistic treatment. Naturopathists are usually trained in a variety of disciplines such as acupuncture, herbalism, homeopathy, osteopathy, hydrotherapy, massage and nutritional therapy.

The modern concept of naturopathy stems from 19th-century Germany where practitioners believed that almost any disease or disorder could be cured by natural means, particularly by diet, fresh air, sunlight and exercise. They also paid particular attention to intestinal and bowel health as a way of keeping the body clean. In Germany today, practitioners are licensed by the state and are highly popular.

Like many complementary therapies, naturopathy is based on the belief that the body has the innate power to heal itself. This power, the life force, helps maintain a healthy equilibrium (homeostasis) which can be weakened by an unhealthy lifestyle such as poor diet, stress, drinking to excess and so on. All of these allow toxins or waste to build up in the body, and the system then becomes unbalanced and more vulnerable to allergies or infection. So, for example, a naturopath might look for lifestyle factors which may have caused a lower sperm count, hormonal imbalance or high blood pressure. They may use a variety of diagnostic tools including iridology (the examination of the eyes to diagnose health conditions), hair analysis and testing muscle strength.

Treatment falls into two main categories, catabolic or cleansing, which may include fasting to help detoxification, and anabolic or strengthening, which aims to build up a weakened constitution by good nutrition and supplements. Treatments vary according to individuals – both practitioners and patients – but the following list gives an idea of what to expect if you consult a naturopath.

- If the naturopath feels the sex hormones are unbalanced, you may be advised not to eat meat from cattle fattened on oestrogen, as this may further unbalance the sex hormones and so result in loss of desire; organic meat or a vegetarian diet might be suggested instead.

- In cases of erectile dysfunction caused by poor blood flow, specific dietary measures may be suggested to help protect the heart, such as oily fish, garlic and ginger.
- Men with impotence might also be given advice on skin brushing with a soft brush or loofah to help improve circulation and eliminate waste.

Dr Dean Ornish, an American physician, has developed a successful naturopathic programme for prevention of and recovery from heart disease, a common underlying cause of impotence in men.

- If you are a northern European or American man, or if you have moved to these parts of the world, acknowledge the possibility of cardiovascular disease.
- As a matter of urgency, adopt activities which encourage the expression of emotions, such as painting or writing poetry or singing in a choir.
- Eat fruit and vegetables at the start of meals every day.
- Avoid fatty foods and those which have been cooked in re-fried oil.
- If you are a smoker, consider giving up.
- Drink alcohol only with meals.
- Have massage and learn how to massage.

All these points concur with many of the other therapies and lifestyle suggestions in this book, and can only benefit physical and emotional health in general.

Numerology

Numerology has been used for many purposes, from winning a lover to helping childless couples conceive, and is based on the concept that the universe is constructed in a mathematical pattern. According to this, all things may be expressed in numbers. 'The world is built upon the power of numbers' is a saying credited to the Greek mathamatician Pythagoras, claimed as the father of numerology because of his discovery that musical intervals as he knew them could be expressed in ratios between the numbers 1, 2, 3 and 4. Each primary number is supposed to have certain characteristics and a male or female aspect. Odd numbers are masculine, creative and active, while even numbers are said to be feminine and passive.

Numerologists believe that one's name is the expression of the universe's vibrations at the time of one's birth, which determines character and destiny. Every letter of your name (vowels and consanants) has a numerical value. Add them together and you will find the number which influences your personality and influences your fate. Specific numbers are believed to have specific attributes when it comes to romance and sex. This analysis is also used by some numerologists to discover which karmic lessons the individual has to face in life. For example, a 2 might indicate the need to focus on details in relationships. Changing your name can alter your destiny, but it may take months or years for the vibratory pattern to change.

Numerologists believe that all words relevant to your life can be converted to numbers to see what could be complementing or blocking your life – your city or street name, for example, as well as your career or your partner's name. Numerology can also be used as a guide for health and for selecting your partner and friends. Some Arab numerologists believe that certain numbers are friendly or amicable – if you carve one on a piece of fruit and hand it to your would-be lover, and he or she eats it, you can hope for success. The number 5 is said to be the number for sensuality and pleasure.

For more details, see Further Reading.

Reflexology

Foot massage is very relaxing and some people may find it enjoyably sensuous. However, reflexology is rather more than this, and is said to be a modern revival of an ancient healing technique used in China, India and Egypt. Like many other natural therapists, reflexologists believe that the body is a dynamic energy field. Reflexology works along the same lines as acupuncture in that reflexologists believe that lines of this energy, chi, run through the body along twelve meridian pathways. The six main meridians that penetrate the major organs of the body are found in the feet, which can be 'mapped' with specific 'zones' corresponding to different parts of the body. Massaging these meridian pathways helps clear blockages along the meridians and encourages the vital body energy to flow. Whether it's a question of easing tension and strain which can impair perfomance, encouraging sexual energy, balancing sexual hormones or working on other conditions which may be interfering with sexual expression, reflexogy can be used therapeutically to treat a wide range of conditions.

THE REPRODUCTIVE REFLEXES

All the reproductive organ reflexes are found around the ankle area, and are as follows (see Figure 5).

Outer ankle – ovaries/testes reflex

Inner ankle – uterus, prostate, vagina and penis

1 *To work on the uterus or prostate reflexes.* (See Figure 6.) These are on the inner foot below the ankle bone. To pinpoint the exact area, place the tip of your index finger on the ankle bone and the tip of your ring finger on the back corner of the heel. Now, with the middle finger, find the middle point between the two in a straight line. The area you need to work on is around the size of a large coin.

   Support the foot in one of your cupped hands and work with the other, using your thumb in what's called the 'rotating thumb technique'. (See Figure 7.) Bend your thumb a little and press gently into the foot with its tip, being careful not to dig in to the flesh with your nail. Rotate your thumb clockwise or anticlockwise, using firm, constant pressure.

2 *To work on the ovaries or testes reflex.* (See Figure 8.) These are below the outside ankle bone. Locate the exact spot using the technique described above.

   Use the same thumb technique and work below the outside of the ankle bone, covering the entire area. (See Figure 9.)

These exercises will help stimulate and balance the hormones that control sexual desire in women and men. They may be used to boost desire, or a reflexologist may also use them therapeutically to work on more obstinate cases of sexual dysfunction, perhaps in combination with other areas which reflect other parts of the body. You can try the

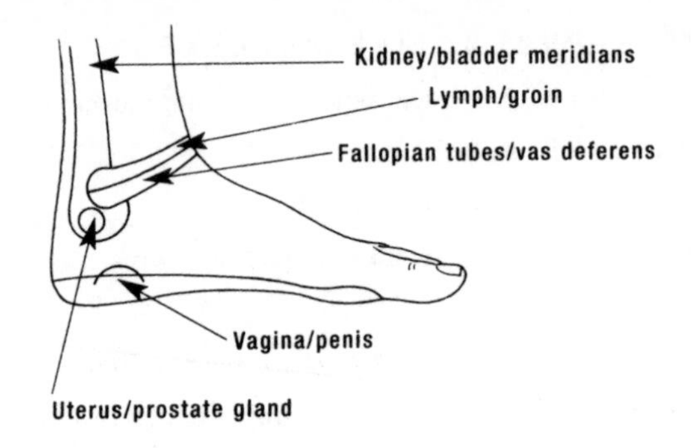

5 The reproductive organ reflexes.

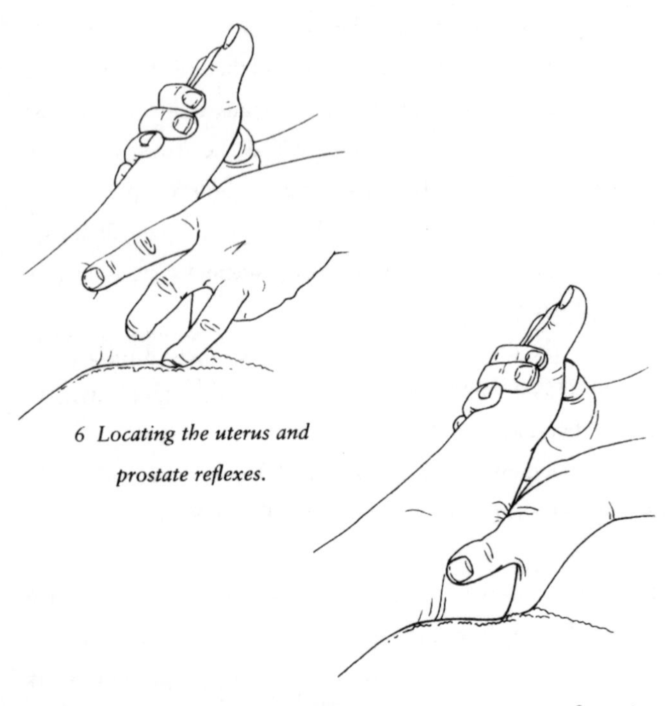

6 Locating the uterus and prostate reflexes.

7 Working the uterus/prostate reflex using the rotating thumb technique.

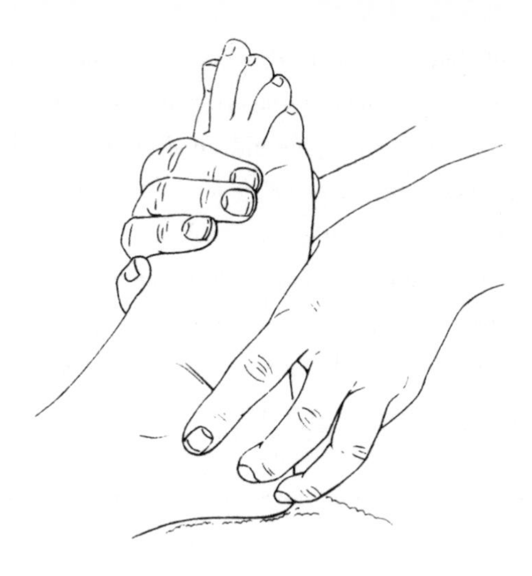

8 Locating the ovaries and testes reflexes.

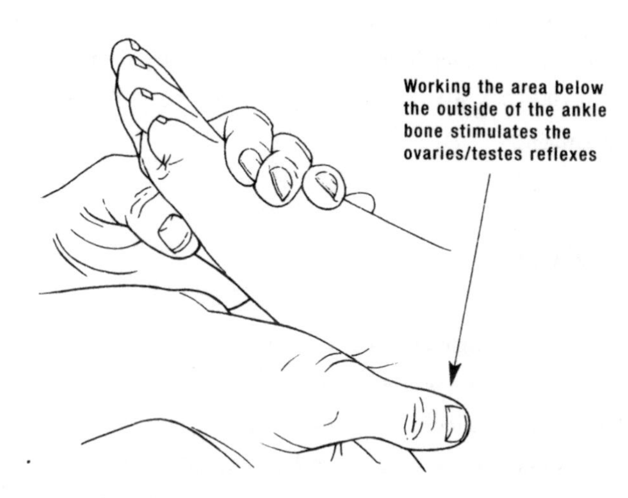

9 Working the ovaries/testes reflex using the rotating thumb technique.

exercises yourself, but you might also like to consult a qualified reflexologist for a proper diagnosis and effective treatment.

A reflexology treatment is a highly indvidual affair depending on your own unique state of health, made up of a combination of factors, and before actually starting work, a reflexologist will talk through your medical history with you in order to decide on the most effective approach. Some people do feel sensitive about subjecting their feet to treatment, perhaps through embarrassment at their size or shape, or because they can't bear having their feet touched. But a reflexology session is usually pleasant and relaxing, and the therapist will apply firm enough pressure for it not to tickle and set up sensitive reactions!

After the treatment, reactions can vary – you may want to go home and sleep for hours, or you may experience a range of emotional reactions such as depression and weepiness. Adverse physical reactions can happen too, such as headaches, aggravated skin conditions or outbreaks of a disease which has been suppressed. This is considered to be a normal, even desirable, part of the healing process and shows the body is ridding itself of toxins. You can help the process along by drinking 6–8 glasses of mineral or warm, boiled water after a treatment.

Shiatsu

Shiatsu, the Japanese for finger pressure, is a healing art originating in Japan which uses the power of touch to enable the body to get in touch with its own self-healing abilities. Shiatsu involves massage (by elbow, knee and heel as well as fingers!) at certain points on the body to induce a feeling of deep relaxation and wellbeing which can certainly be enough to help with loss of libido induced by stress and emotional tension.

Shiatsu is said to access the 12 channels ('meridians') where the life energy, *qi* or *chi* (in Chinese), *ki* (in Japanese), flows through the body. The meridians are said to influence different organs and body systems.

Shiatsu practitioners believe that when energy becomes blocked, the body may produce physical symptoms or psychological or emotional disturbances. Shiatsu uses physical pressure to unblock these areas so that the energy can flow freely again. And, by focusing on the *kyo*, the hidden or underlying cause of disease, Shiatsu may be used to treat both milder cases of loss of desire, and more deep-rooted, long-term cases of sexual dysfunction, as well as any other health problems which underly them. For example, because Shiatsu works on the body's inner organs as well as the skin and muscles, Shiatsu can be used to treat circulatory problems which may play a part in erectile difficulties.

DIY SHIATSU MASSAGE

You can try the following two massages yourself, or ask a partner to do them.

The Sea of Intimacy

Use light pressure and work with your fingertips or palm placed gently on the skin, as you will be working on sensitive areas which people are not used to having touched. This exercise is said to stimulate the kidney meridian, believed to be linked with sexuality.

- Place one hand over the other on the abdomen on the so-called Sea of Intimacy points located two, three and four finger widths below the navel.

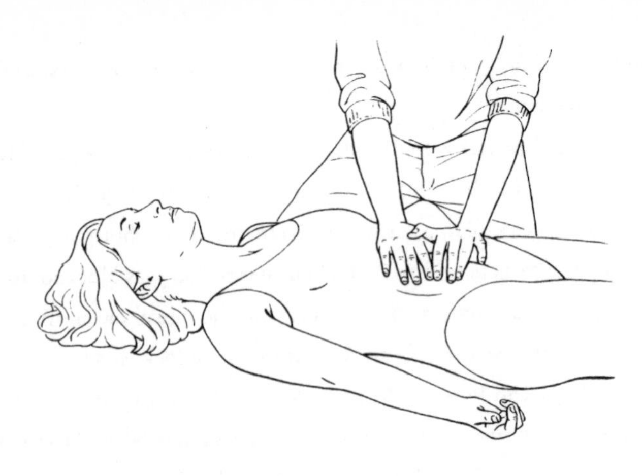

10 The Sea of Intimacy Shiatsu massage.

- Keeping your hands in place, slowly rock your body backward and forward so that the hands move gently back and forth on the abdomen, a bit like kneading dough gently (see Figure 10). Don't rub, but keep your hands lightly placed on the same area of skin.
- Keep this up for three minutes. Be sure to end gently.

Centring the head

Many important meridians begin and end in the head, which along with the neck is an area where many people tend to hold much of their energy. You probably know yourself how a stiffly-held head and tight neck are key signs of retained tension. In particular, one of the meridians, the Governing Vessel, runs centrally from the spine to the crown and the forehead before going deep into the body. The Governing Vessel is said to be associated with sexual disorders and lack of vitality.

Again, use light pressure and work just with your fingertips.

- To centre the head, place one thumb on top of the other just above the point between the eyebrows.
- Gently work up the centre of the forehead to the top of the crown using fingertips in a light massage.
- You could terminate this exercise with a light finger massage all over the head and down to the base of the skull where the neck area begins. This is very refreshing and relaxing.

ACUPRESSURE POINTS

Shiatsu is a Japanese interpretation of acupressure, a Chinese discipline directly descended from acupuncture. Instead of using needles, however, acupressure uses pressure, usually with the thumb, to the relevant point. Acupressure is easy to do at home, though you may need the help of your partner or another friend to reach the points which are located down your back as described in the exercises below.

Massage with your thumb, working slowly and carefully, without jabbing. Aim to press into the skin until you feel resistance, but not so as to cause pain. The following points are recommended for treating impotence and lack of desire.

- Bladder meridian 22 – level with the lower portion of the first lumbar vertebra (see Figure 11).
- Bladder meridian 23 – level with the space between the second and third lumbar vertebrae (see Figure 11).
- Conception Vessel meridian 4 – on the midline of the abdomen, four fingers' width below the navel (see Figure 12).
- Conception Vessel meridian 7 – on the midline of the abdomen, onethumb's width below the navel (see Figure 12).

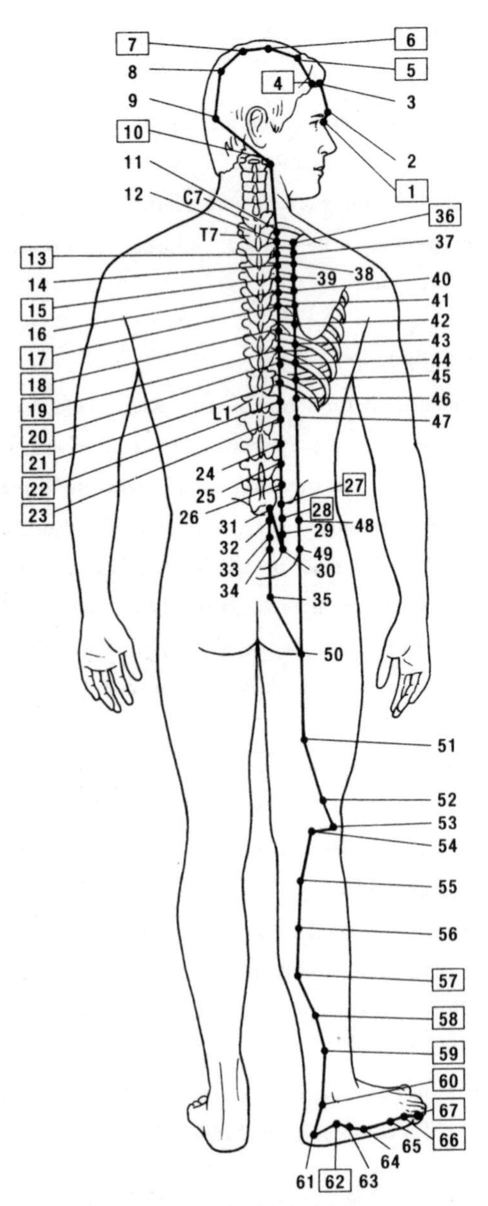

11 The bladder meridian.

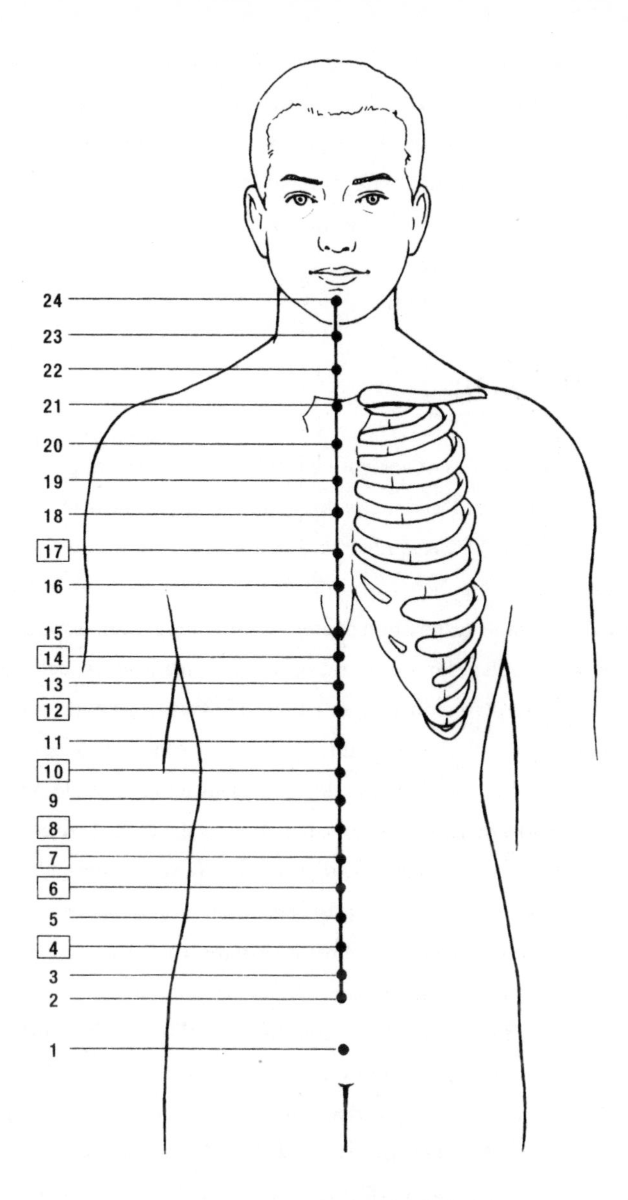

12 The conception vessel meridian.

The last two are the same points as the Sea of Intimacy point mentioned above in the DIY Shiatsu massage, but you are using a different massage technique, i.e. the thumb instead of the whole hand. Some people find this more effective but if you are sensitive in this area you might find the gentle kneading technique better as described under 'The Sea of Intimacy'.

Tai chi chuan

Tai chi chuan is a series of ancient Chinese exercises used to promote health and vitality, induce inner calm and improve the flow of *chi* or the life force. A 1996 UK study found that blood pressure was lower in post-heart-attack patients who practice tai chi, so it may be able to help with erectile dysfunction caused by poor circulation. Research indicates that it relaxes muscles and nerves, benefits posture, balance and flexibility and can reduce stress symptoms. Two American studies have found it helps with stress and improves breathing efficiency.

Tai chi is based on the Taoist philosophy of living in harmony with nature. Some adherents like to work barefoot on the earth in order to be in touch with nature's energy – what is called 'breathing through the feet'. This is based on the works of the great Taoist philosopher Chuang Tzu (c. 200BC) who said that, 'The breathing of the true man comes from his heels, while men generally breathe only from their throats.' The earliest type of tai chi seems to have been practised around 1700BC, when Huang Ti, the Yellow Emperor, practised a form of exercise called Daoyin (*dao* means guide and *yin* means leading) in order to gain longevity. The exercises combined breathing techniques with body movements designed to increase circulation and flush toxins out of the body. Through this kind of exercise combined with meditation, Huang Ti is said to have reigned for 100 years, during which time he also had several wives.

Said also to have been practised by Taoist monks in the 13th century, tai chi has also been promoted by the Chinese government as a form of preventative health care, and this is one of its main uses – to prevent fatigue and raise energy, rather than cure established disorders or diseases. Tai chi is supposed to encourage the flow of chi through the body. Chi exists as yang, a masculine energy, and yin, a female energy, both of which must be in harmony for health and happiness. Yang is pulled down from the skies, while yin is pulled up through the earth through breathing techniques. The practice of tai chi gradually dissolves energy blockages within the body and between the body and its environment; as a result, overall health balance is better. It also forms an effective spiritual and mental discipline, as well as a non-combative martial art for self-defence. There are five major styles: Chen, Yang, Wu, Woo and Sun. Yang, the most common in the West, is a rhythmical series of slowly performed postures.

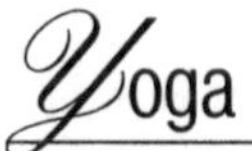oga

A powerful way of reducing stress, yoga combines breathing, relaxation and meditation as well as stretching and massaging inner organs. It was developed many thousands of years ago as a scientific method enabling its practitioners to develop physically, mentally and psychologically into more complete human beings. Hatha yoga, the type most commonly practised in the West, focuses on physical exercises, or asanas. The syllables *ha* and *tha* mean the sun and moon, or the flux of positive and negative energies. Balance of these energies results in health, imbalance in disease. Each posture is designed to have specific effects on certain parts of the body, and some of the asanas can be used to boost libido as well as working on related problems such as circulation. This all takes place as part of a general boost to fitness and energy. Correct use of the asanas can hep eliminate toxins, revitalize the body and strengthen the entire nervous system. In addition, by stimulating endocrine activity, Hatha yoga can help regulate emotions, so leaving you with a calmer, clearer mind.

BEFORE STARTING

- If you have any existing physical problems or illnesses, or if you are in any doubt at all as to whether you should do yoga, consult your doctor.
- It helps to do the exercises at around the same time each day. You may find that morning is a good time for alertness, or the exercises may help you relax in the evening.
- You should wait two hours after a main meal, and one hour after a snack. Try not to eat for half an hour after exercising.
- Wear light comfortable clothing and practise barefoot if possible. Remove jewellery or other items which could be a hazard.
- It can help to take a warm bath before doing the exercises, especially if you are not naturally flexible.
- Warming up is important to prime your muscles for the asanas, or poses, and in order to avoid muscle strain, so spend some time gently stretching or doing light exercises before each session.
- When doing the asanas, only hold the position for as long as is comfortable, even if that's just a second or two. You should not have to strain to achieve a posture, and certainly should not experience any pain (if you do, stop immediately).
- Never rush, and keep your movements slow and steady.

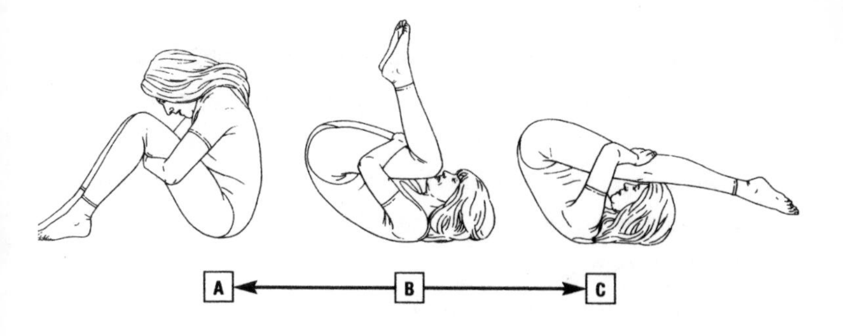

13 Rocking the spine.

- Spend time relaxing afterwards – sitting quietly, or lying covered with a light blanket – either by yourself or with your partner.

WARM-UP EXERCISES

- Slowly rotate your shoulders first backwards and then forwards a few times. This deceptively simple exercise helps keep the shoulders and upper back area relaxed – a prime area for tension build-up.
- Try Rocking the Spine (see Figure 13 at a, b and c) to stimulate circulation, massage your spine, and give you a surge of energy. Sit with your legs bent and clasp your hands under your knees (Figure 13a). Keeping your head low to your knees, rock backwards and forwards (Figure 13b). Once you feel comfortable with this, rock backwards right onto your back (Figure 13c). If possible, get your toes to touch the floor, or as far as they will go, but do not force the posture. Rocking the Spine can also be used for those with back pain, but, if in doubt as to whether you should do yoga with a bad back, do consult your doctor first.

POSTURES (ASANAS)

Rooster

This standing pose is easy to perform, helps effective breathing, boosts energy, and is said to be an effective sexual energizer (see Figure 14).

1 Stand straight with your feet close together. Make sure your back is held straight but not stiff, and that your arms are held down with the palms of your hands held outward (Figure 14a).
2 Breathe in deeply, blowing your abdomen outwards while lifting your arms and touching your fingers together above your head (Figure 14b).
3 Now pull your tummy in and breath out, while slowly lowering your arms to your sides.
4 Lift yourself on to your toes and breathe in, holding your arms out at either side. Breathe freely and balance for a few seconds (Figure 14c).

Repeat three times.

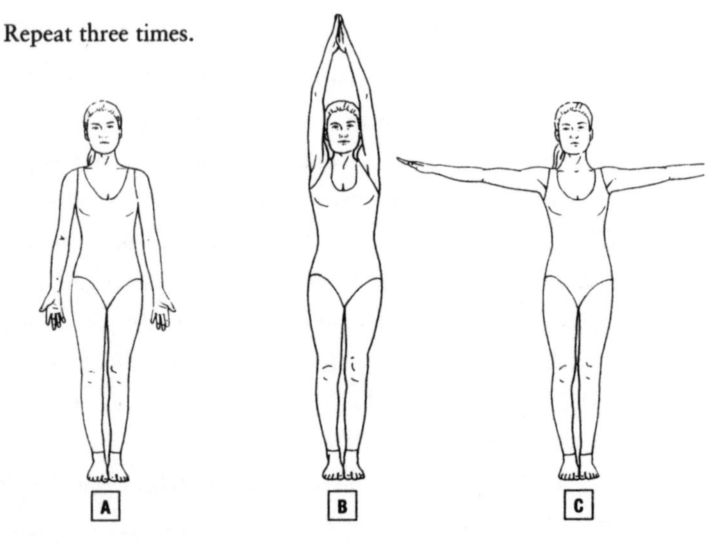

14 The Rooster.

Camel

Be sure to warm up before doing this one and if your spine is stiff, be careful to bend back only as far as is comfortable to avoid strain. The Camel is good for the internal organs within the abdomen and helps circulation, and may also help boost low libido (see Figure 15).

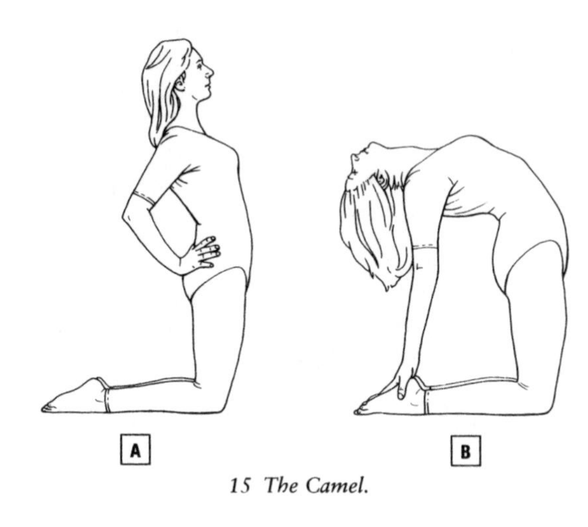

15 The Camel.

1 Kneel with legs apart and hands on your hips (Figure 15a). Bend slightly backward while breathing in. Hold for five seconds or as long as you can. Breathe out and return to the upright kneeling position.
2 Breathe in and bend right backward, reaching for your heels or ankles (Figure 15b). Breathe freely and hold for 5–10 seconds. Breathe out and slowly raise yourself up to the kneeling position.

Repeat three times.

Shoulderstand

The shoulderstand (see Figure 16) is a wonderful all-purpose energizer: it tones the endocrine glands, improves circulation, combats stress and is even supposed to help keep you young and beautiful!

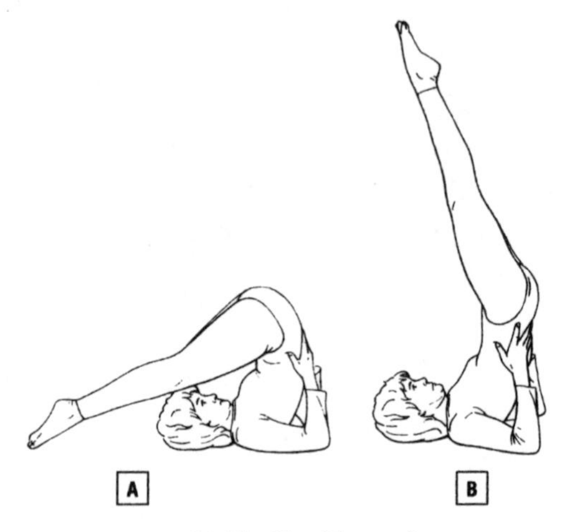

16 The Shoulderstand.

1 Lie flat on your back with your legs together and your arms at your sides.
2 Breathe in and raise your legs up and as far as possible over your head. Use your hands to support your back, placing them just above the buttocks. Keep your legs straight and close together if possible (Figure 16a).
3 Still supporting your back with your hands, push your legs right up so they are vertical (Figure 16b). The weight of your body should be on your shoulders and arms. If you cannot manage to keep your legs straight, hold them bent at the knees or whichever angle you find most comfortable.

4 Hold the pose for 30–60 seconds.
5 Lower yourself back down gently, using abdominal muscles to avoid creating tension in the shoulders.
6 Relax completely in a lying position.

Repeat two or three times.

Wonderful water

Water is a powerful therapy: it is a beautifier, booster and cleanser. Traditionally, it has been used in all sorts of cultures for all sorts of benefits. Water can be used in a number of ways. You can apply it to parts of the body; bathe part or all of yourself in it; add substances such as oils or salts to help its effects. You can also exercise in it, and because you float, you can often achieve much more in water than on dry land! What's more, it's cheap, enjoyable and easy to do, especially at home. Water therapy can, in particular, help boost circulation, and so aid effective sexual performance. Warm or hot water causes muscles to relax and blood vessels to open or dilate (much the same action as Viagra, in fact!) so causing more blood to reach the relevant tissues. Cold water has the opposite effect, contracting blood vessels, which decongests and clears the tissues; and, when hot water is applied afterwards, the tissues are flushed with fresh, oxygen-rich blood.

THERMO-REGULATORY HYDROTHERAPY

Research at London's Brompton Hospital showed that cold baths bring a number of benefits including a boost in sex hormone production, which helps regulate potency in men and and women, renewed energy and improved circulation. The treatment used was Thermo-Regulatory Hydrotherapy (TRH), and internationally renowned naturopath and author Leon Chaitow (see Further Reading) recommends the following sequence in this four-stage process (which might be fun to try with a partner!).

Do follow the stages in the order given as it is essential that the body is 'trained' towards a good response. Have the bath water as cold as you can bear it – between 54.9°F and 65°F (12.7°C and 18.3°C).

1. Stand in cold water in the bath for 3–5 minutes, either walking up and down or marching on the spot. Be sure to use a non-slip mat. Continue this stage daily for 10 days in order to condition the body.
2. Sit in cold water for another 3–5 minutes – the pooled blood in the lower part of the body cools and further influences the hypothalamus, which influences the release of the sexual hormones. Continue this stage daily for two to three weeks.
3. This is the most important part of the programme. Immerse your entire body up to the neck and back of the head in cold water, moving your arms and legs gently to ensure that the cooling process is evenly spread over your body. Stay in the bath for 10–20 minutes. Continue daily.
4. This is the 're-warming stage'. Give yourself a brisk rub-down with a towel and then exercise for a minute or two, skipping or running on the spot. This should produce a warm glow. Continue daily.

Caution: Do not undertake TRH if you have a heart condition, high blood pressure or chronic disease requiring regular prescription medication. Consult your doctor first.

SITZ BATHS

If a candle-lit bath scented by a few drops of your favourite oil doesn't do the trick, you might want to try a more drastic remedy. Cold baths come from a long line of European hydrotherapy techniques, and have been recommended for impotence. Alternating hot and cold sitz baths, a technique which can easily be used at home, increase the circulation of blood to the pelvic area and improve vitality. The idea is to place the pelvic area (buttocks and hips up to the navel) in water at one temperature, while your feet are placed in water of the same or contrasting temperature. Certain parts of the body, when heated or cooled, have a reflex effect on the circulation of more distant areas – the skin on the feet (and hands) has a reflex connection to the pelvic region and especially the reproductive organs, which means that heating or cooling hands or feet should have an impact on the reproductive area.

- 1–3 minutes seated in hot water (106–110°F/41–43°C)
- 15–30 seconds in cold (around 60°F/15°C)
- 1–3 minutes hot
- 15 seconds cold.

While immersing your hips, try to have your feet in water of a contrasting temperature, so that when your hips are in hot water, your feet are in cold and vice versa – but if this is difficult to do, then just go for the hip immersion. Afterwards, you might like to wrap yourself (or selves) in a big, warm towel, without drying yourself, and lie down for at least 10 minutes.

Caution: Do not try this treatment if you have heart problems, bladder or kidney problems, or suffer from haemorrhage, colic or spasm.

DRINK IT!

Water is one of most vital dietary needs though most people tend to disregard or forget it. We are made up of 60 per cent water. Drinking enough water helps you mentally and physically in many ways – for example it helps you feel more alert, keeps your digestion ticking over, cleanses the colon and digestive tract, is good for the skin, and may help you lose weight. Don't drink it in the form of tea or coffee as these are diurectic and just make your kidneys work harder.

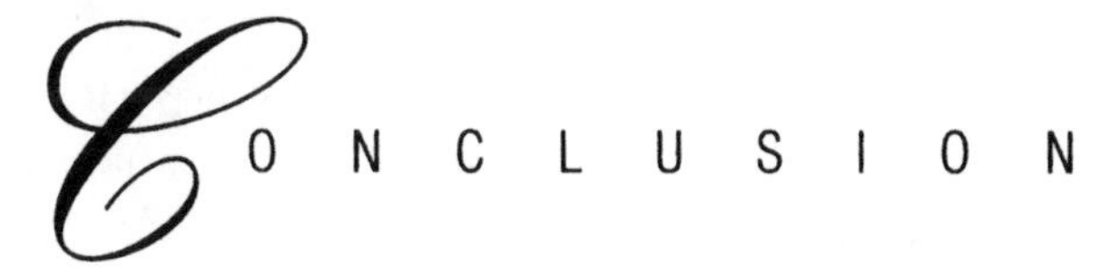

CONCLUSION

SEX is often viewed as a kind of spontaneous combustion – a vast force beyond conscious control, which simply happens and takes the participants over. Or should do! If it doesn't, it's easy to think that something must surely be wrong. But, after looking through this book, we can see how sexuality is formed from many differing components which make up the whole, just as many different parts make up the whole body. Sexuality is not really a separate entity which we can hold up and show people; it is an attitude, a perspective and a reflection of our health or of the way we view ourselves.

This inner perspective can change if we alter any of the components which make it up. After reading this book, I hope you will realize how simple it can be to enjoy a better quality of sex by purposely changing areas of your life. Being more aware of how your sexuality functions doesn't mean that spontaneity will be lost. On the contrary, being in peak physiological, emotional and spiritual health means that you will find it easier to let go and enjoy sexual expression on your terms than ever before.

A major step towards improvement is acceptance. This really means acceptance of your own individuality. While many have danced the sexual dance before you, only you can really know how you feel, and what you hope for. Once you have recognized and accepted the gap betwen expectation and reality, you can proceed on the way forward.

Hopefully, reading this book will have given you plenty of ideas which you can start putting into practice immediately. Some people may prefer to experiment by themselves as the mood takes them to see which remedies they find most effective, for example trying out a detox treatment when they feel off-colour. To help you follow up areas of interest discussed in this book, an extensive list of books is recommended in the 'Further Reading' section.

If you decide you want to consult a practitioner, either after a period of experimenting or at once, the choice is wide. Some specialist addresses are also given at the end of this book in the 'Useful Addresses' section. Many of these will be able to give you names and addresses of practitioners in your area. Other options are to look in your local telephone directory, on your local library noticeboard or to explore research options such as the internet. Probably better still is to ask around – at your health food store, perhaps at an exercise class you attend, or via a friend. However, while word of mouth is an effective way of meeting a practitioner of integrity, personal recommendation doesn't necessarily mean that the treatment will be right for you. Sex being the delicate interpersonal beast it is, finding a practitioner with whom you feel comfortable is really important, so, if necessary, take the time to investigate the different options before committing yourself to a course of treatment.

Alternative holidays are a growing area for those who feel they would like to extend their interest further, or to explore therapies in more detail than is possible in the stress and bustle of everyday life. For example, one company offers yoga holidays in the Canary Islands; another, naturopathy holidays on the Aegean island of Skyros (again, see Useful Addresses). Alternative holidays offer a programme of activities and therapies which aim to help people 'escape' in the deepest sense, so that they can return to ordinary life with a fresh vision and sense of purpose. This can be especially valuable in dealing with the tensions which can escalate from unsatisfactory sexual performance. Health farms are another option for those who would perhaps just like a weekend break in order to detox. Ask your travel agent, or again try researching via the internet.

Regaining your sexuality can be a rewarding quest, often in subtle and unforeseen ways. It may lead you along novel paths, transform your attitudes and enrich your quality of life well beyond your original expectations. In chaos theory, it is said that a butterfly fluttering its wings in Japan will have reverberations throughout the world. Likewise, tackling this very central area of life may reverberate on your entire individual cosmos, too!

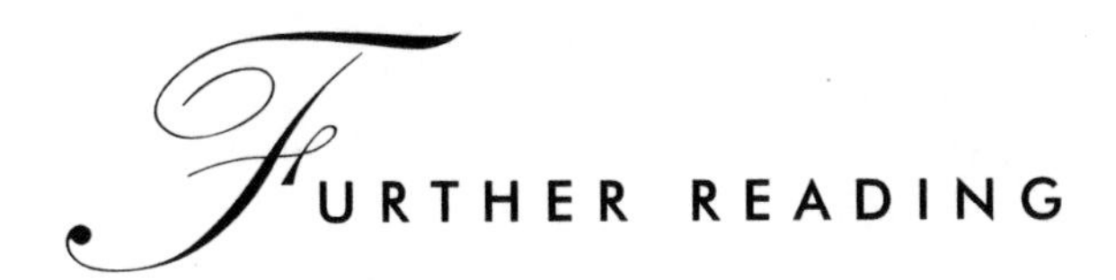

FURTHER READING

Brennan, Richard, *The Alexander Technique*, Vega, 2002

Brewer, Sarah, *The Comlpete Book of Men's Health*, Thorsons, 1995

Brewer, Sarah, *Better Sex*, Marshall Publishing, 1995

Campion, Kitty, *Holistic Woman's Herbal*, Bloomsbury, 1997

Carr, Rachel, *Yoga for All Ages*, Simon & Schuster, 1972

Carroll, Steve, *The Which? Guide to Men's Health*, Consumer's Association, 1997

Cowmeadow, Oliver, *Shiatsu, A Practical Introduction*, Element Books, 1998

Davis, Adelle, *Let's Get Well*, Unwin, 1983

Ducie, Sonia, *Do It Yourself Numerology*, Element Books, 1998

Farquharson, Marie, *Natural Detox*, Vega, 2001

Fraser, James, *The Golden Bough, a study in magic and religion*, (1890); reprint Chancellor Press, 1994

Herbert, Lauren, *Sex and Back Pain*, available only in the US on 00 1 207 695 3354

Kent, Howard, *Breathe Better Feel Better*, Apple Press, 1998

Kirkwood, Tom, *Time of Our Lives*, Weidenfeld & Nicolson 1999

Lad, Vasant, *The Complete Book of Ayurvedic Home Remedies*, Piatkus, 1999

Lamm, Steven MD, *Younger at Last*, Simon & Schuster, 1997

Lindenfield, Gael, *Assert Yourself*, Thorsons, 1987

Lindenfield, Gael, *Managing Anger*, Thorsons, 1993

Mann, John, *Murder, Magic, and Medicine*, Oxford University Press, 1994

McIntyre, Michael, *Herbal Medicine for Everyone, A guide to the theory and practice of herbal medicine*, Arkana, 1990

Shealy, C. Norman, *The Illustrated Encyclopaedia of Healing Remedies*, Element Books, 1998

Tobyn, Graeme, *Culpeper's Medicine, A practice of Western Holistic Medicine*, Element Books, 1997

Weller, Stella, *The Yoga Back Book*, Thorsons, 1993

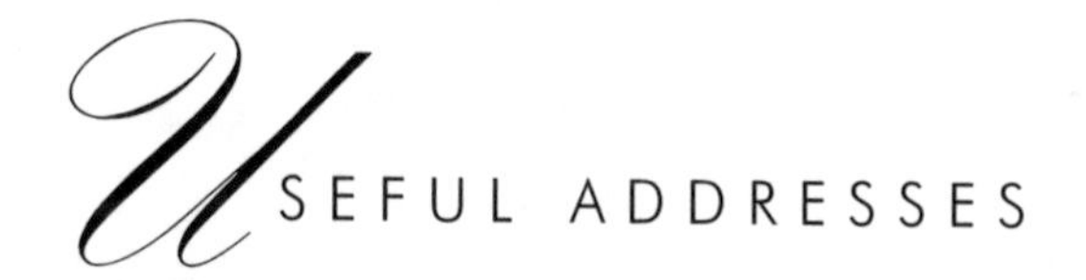

USEFUL ADDRESSES

ALEXANDER TECHNIQUE

Australia
Alexander Technique International, 11/11 Stanley St, Darlinghurst, NSW 2010

Canada
The Canadian Society of Teachers of the Alexander Technique, Box 47025, Apt 12 555 West 12th Avenue, Vancouver, BC, V5Z 3XO

Europe and UK
The Society of Teachers of the Alexander Technique, 20 London House, 266 Fulham Road, London SW10 9EL

Alexander Technique International, 66c Thurlestone Road, London SE27 0PD

USA
The North American Society of Teachers of the Alexander Technique, PO Box 112484, Tacoma, WA 98411-2484

AROMATHERAPY

Australia
International Federation of Aromatherapists, 1/390 Burwood Road, Hawthorn BIC3122. Tel: 039530 0067

Europe and UK
Aromatherapy Organizations Council, PO Box 355, Croydon CR9 2QP. Tel/Fax: 0208 251 7912

Aromatherapy Organizations Council, 3 Latimer Close, Braybrooke, Market Harborough, Leicester LE16 8LN

International Federation of
Aromatherapists,
Stamford House,
182 Chiswick High Road,
London W4 1PP.
Tel: 0208 742 2605
Fax: 0208 742 2606

International Federation of
Professional Aromatherapists,
82 Ashby Road, Hinckley,
Leicester LE10 1SN.
Tel: 0145 637 987

South Africa
Association of Aromatherapists,
PO Box 23924,
Claremont 7735.
Tel: 021 531 297

USA
American Alliance of
Aromatherapy,
PO Box 750428,
Petaluma,
California 94975-0428

American Aromatherapy
Association,
PO Box 3679,
South Pasadena,
California 91031

ART THERAPY

The Institute for Arts in Therapy
and Education,
Windsor Centre,
Windsor Street,
London N1 8QG.
Tel: 0207 704 2534

AYURVEDA

Australia
Maharishi Ayurveda Health
Centres,
PO Box 81, Bundoora,
Victoria 3083

Europe and UK
Ayurvedic Company of
Great Britain,
50 Penywern Road,
London SW5 9XS

Ayurvedic Living,
PO Box 188, Exeter,
Devon EX4 5AB

Ayurvedic Medical Association UK,
The Hale Clinic, 7 Park Crescent,
London W1N 3HE

Eastern Clinic,
1079 Garret Lane, Tooting,
London SW17 0LN
Tel: 0208 682 3876

South Africa
South African Ayurvedic Medicine Association,
85 Harvey Road,
Morningside, Durban 4001.
Tel: 031 303 3245

USA
American Holistic Medical Association,
6728 McLean Village Drive,
McLean, VA 22101-8729

The Ayurvedic Institute,
Dr Vasant Lad,
11311 Menaul NE,
Albuquerque,
New Mexico 87112.
Tel: 505 291 9698

The Ayurveda Institute,
PO Box 282, Fairfield,
Iowa 52556.
Tel: 310 454 5531

International Federation for Ayurveda, Ayurvedic Medicine of New York,
Scott Gerson MD,
13 West Ninth Street,
New York, NY 10011.
Tel: 212 505 8971

BREATHWORK

International Breathwork Foundation.
Tel: 0845 4581050

HERBALISM (WESTERN AND CHINESE)

Australia
National Herbalists Association of Australia, Suite 305,
BST House, 3 Small Street,
Broadway,
NSW 2007.
Tel: 02 211 6437

Chinese and Herbal Centre,
2392–2394 Sussex Street,
Sydney, NSW 2000

Canada
Canadian Natural Health Association,
439 Wellington Street, Toronto,
Ontario M5V 2H7.
Tel: 416 977 2642

Europe and UK
General Council and Register of Consultant Herbalists,
18 Sussex Square, Brighton,
East Sussex BN2 5AA

National Institute of Medical Herbalists,
56 Longbrooke Street,
Exeter EX4 8HA

Register of Chinese Herbal Medicine,
21 Warbreck Road,
London W10 8NS

South Africa
South African Naturopaths and Herbalists Association,
PO Box 18663,
Wynberg 7824

The Herb Society of South Africa,
PO Box 37721,
Overport

USA
American Herbalists Guild,
1931 Gaddis Road,
Canton,
CA 30115.
Tel: 770 751 6021

American Association of Oriental Medicine,
5530 Wisconsin Avenue,
Suite 1210,
Chevy Chase,
MD 20815.
Tel: 888 500 7999

HYDROTHERAPY

Europe and UK
The Clarendon Health and Beauty Clinic,
515 Hagley Road,
Birmingham B66 4AX.
Tel: 0121 429 9191

See also address for Naturopathy

MASSAGE

Australia
Association of Massage Therapists,
3/33 Denham Street,
Bondai,
New South Wales, NSW 2026

Europe and UK
Massage Therapy Institute of Great Britain,
PO Box 276,
London NW2 4NR

Massage Training Institute,
24 Highbury Road, London N5.
Tel: 0207 226 5313

USA
American Massage Therapy Association,
820 Davis Street,
Suite 100,
Evanston, Illinois
60201-4444
Tel: 847/864 0123

NATUROPATHY

Canada
Canadian College of
Naturopathic Medicine,
60 Berl Avenue, Toronto,
Ontario M8Y 3CY

UK and Europe
British College of Osteopathic
Medicine,
Lief House,
120 Finchley Road,
London NW3 5HR.
Tel: 0207 435 6464
Fax: 0207 431 3630

USA
American Naturopathic
Association,
1413 King Street,
Washington DC, 20005.
Tel: 202 682 7352

NUMEROLOGY

Australia
Character Analysis and
Numerology,
23 Flinders Street,
Kent Town 5067

UK and Europe
Association Internationale de
Numerologues (AIN),
PO Box 867,
Harrow HA1 3XL

Connaissance School of
Numerology,
Royston Cave,
Art and Book Shop,
8 Melbourne Street,
Royston,
Hertfordshire SG8 7BZ

USA
Marina D. Graham,
7266 Bennett Valley Road,
Santa Rosa,
California 959404-9738

NUTRITION

Canada
National Institute of Nutrition
Suite 302, 265 Carling Avenue,
Ottawa, Ontario K1S 2E1

UK and Europe
Society for the Promotion of
Nutritional Therapy,
http://freespace.virgin.net/
nutrition.therapy

REFLEXOLOGY

UK and Europe
Association of Reflexologists,
27 Old Gloucester Street,
London WCIN 3XX.
Tel: 0870 567 3320

International Institute of
Reflexology,
www.reflexology-uk.net

SEXUAL HEALTH

UK and Europe
London Marriage Guidance
(sexual problems clinic),
76A New Cavendish Street,
London W1M 7LB

Men's Healthline
Tel: 0208 995 4448 (6–10p.m.)

Couples Counselling Service at
St Luke's Hospital for the
Clergy,
London W1T 6AH
Tel: 0207 388 4954

National Relate, Herbert Gray
College, Little Church Street,
Rugby. Tel: 01788 573 241

The Impotence Association
PO Box 10296,
London SW17 9WH.
Helpline: 0208 767 7791

USA
Impotence Information Center,
PO Box 9,
Minneapolis, MN 55440.
Tel: 800 843 4315

Impotence Institute of America,
8201 Corporate Drive,
Suite 320, Landover,
MD 20715.
Tel: 800 669 1603

Sexual Function Health Council,
American Foundation for
Urologic Disease,
1128 North Charles Street,
Baltimore,
MD 21201.
Tel: 410 468 1800

Thc Geddings Osbon, Sr.
Foundation,
PO Drawer 1593,
Augusta, GA 30903-1593.
Tel: 800 433 4215

SHIATSU

UK and Europe
Shiatsu Society,
Eastlands Court,
St Peters Road,
Rugby CV21 3QP.
Tel: 01788 555051
Fax: 01788 555052

USA
American Oriental Bodywork
Therapy Association
(for Shiatsu),
50 Maple Place,
New York, NY 11030

TAI CHI CHUAN

UK
Tai Chi Union for Great Britain,
102 Felsham Road,
London SW15 1DQ

British Tai Chi Chuan
and Shaolin Kung Fu
Association,
28 Linden Farm Drive,
Countesthorpe,
Leicester LE8 3SX

YOGA

Australia
BKS Iyengar Association of
Australia,
PO Box 159,
Mosman, NSW 2088,
Tel: 1 800 677 037

Canada
Sivananda Yoga Vedanta Center,
5178 St Lawrence Boulevard,
Montreal, Quebec H2T 1RB

UK and Europe
British Wheel of Yoga,
25 Jermyn Street,
Sleaford, Lincs NG34 7RU.
Tel: 01529 306851

Yoga for Health Foundation,
Ickwell Bury, Biggleswade,
Bedfordshire SG18 9EF.
Te1: 01767 627271

USA
International Association of
Yoga Therapists,
2400A County Center Drive,
Santa Rosa,
CA 95403.
Tel: 707 566 9000

Sivananda Yoga Vedanta Center,
243 West 24th Street,
New York, NY 10011.
Tel: 212 255 4560

OTHER ADDRESSES

Alternative Holidays
The Skyros Centre, Atsitsa,
Greece, Administration:
92 Prince of Wales Road,
London NW5 3NE.
Tel: 0207 267 4424,
Fax: 0207 284 3063

Human Design
Richard Rudd.
Tel: 01323 870660
email: Merlinus33@aol.com

Yokimbe suppliers
Nutrizec,
PO Box 3102,
Wokingham,
Berkshire RG41 3YW.
Information Helpline:
0118 9619604,
email: jmac@tgis.co.uk

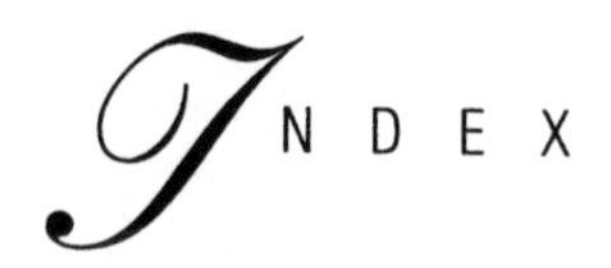

INDEX